MW00576347

KINDLING
WRITINGS ON THE BODY

BY AURORA LEVINS MORALES

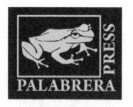

Palabrera Press

Cambridge, Massachusetts

www.palabrerapress.com

© 2013 by Aurora Levins Morales

All rights reserved. No part of this book may be
reproduced or utilized in any form or by any means,
electronic or mechanical, including photocopying,
recording, or any information storage and retrieval system,
without permission in writing from the publisher.

PLEASE RESPECT THE WORKER'S RIGHTS
OF WRITERS AND ARTISTS.

Cover design by Ricardo Levins Morales,
www.rlmartstudio.com

Cover image from 1884 anatomical flipbook published
by L.W. Yaggy, Chicago, courtesy of Ophelia Chong.

Text design by Brittany Rode, Boston, MA

ISBN 9780983683131

Library of Congress Control Number 2013901024

Dedication

There are hundreds of people I could thank, the multitudes who donated money to pay for my attendant care, the attendants who provide that care every day, the team of healers in whom I have the most faith, the friends and family who have provided moral and material support, and I do. I thank them all, with heartfelt gratitude, but here on this page, for this book, I am holding space for the others, the co-sick, the companions of my day to day struggle who lie in their own beds while I lie in mine, sending each other messages, when we have the energy, that bear a special kind of knowing witness to one another. Illness, in spite of the crowds of service providers that surround us, is a solitary state, but thanks to the connecting power of the internet, we throw these messages in bottles into the common sea, fish them out on the tides of pre-dawn pain and afternoon exhaustion, hold each other's stories, cradle them, touch them again and again, these pebbles of experience made silken by the terrible pounding of sickness and poverty, isolation and despair, and a cruel and corrupt profit-driven medical system. Suffering doesn't improve people. It isn't good for us. It isn't intended to inspire. But in the course of it, sometimes the inessential is hacked away, and we become these shining touchstones for each other. So this is for you, mis comadres y compadres. Our stories matter. Our stories ease suffering. Our stories save lives.

Table of Contents

Cuba

Sins Invalid

Introduction

This book was born of desperation. In mid-September of 2012 I began experiencing intense pain in my low back that very quickly became completely disabling, escalating into the worst physical pain I can remember. I have spent the last five months in bed, first dealing with the agony of a pinched nerve, undiagnosed and untreated because when I showed up in the ER on a gurney, the doctor on call gave me three days' worth of narcotics and sent me home, and the primary care doctor assigned to me refused to give me enough medication to make a trip to a doctor's office bearable. I endured under-medicated agonies from the pinched nerve and another set of agonies from the severe constipation the pain medications caused. A month later I finally returned to the ER, on a gurney, and demanded to be admitted, and my pain medications were increased. I am now in the middle of a long, slow process of withdrawing from opiates I became dependent on. I still have enough back pain to keep me from sitting at my desk or walking to the corner. I still spend most of my time in bed. I'm trying to get the Pain Clinic I have a referral to, to be scent free enough so I can tolerate getting care. Every physical therapist who has come to the house has reeked of chemicals that make me very sick.

During the early months, I had to wear diapers because the pain was so bad, I was unable to roll over, let alone get out of bed to sit on a commode. I live with my 82 year old father, who, much as he loves me, can't take care of me himself, and for much of this time I've needed round the clock attendants. The cost of hiring them ourselves comes to $11,000 a month. We used up all of my savings in the first month.

Because I live in a rich country whose health care system is controlled by corporations, for profit, not public health, and whose policy makers, at the service of private wealth, not collective wellness, have been systematically slashing budgets and closing doors, there is no social safety cushion for me.

I have been chronically ill for most of my life, though I didn't know it. I thought my constant state of exhaustion was a character defect, a lack of willpower, perhaps laziness or a dislike of working. In spite of the fact that strove, constantly, to invent livelihoods for myself, in spite of my good radical upbringing, and the sure knowledge that poverty is systemic and deliberate, I thought it was my fault.

In fact, I inherited nine malfunctioning liver enzymes that interfere with my body's ability to clean up and expel toxins, had heavy pesticide exposure as a young child, developed epilepsy, possibly as a result, and experienced intensely traumatic sexual and psychological abuse at the hands of a ring of traffickers connected to my grade school. My seizures have resulted in multiple brain injuries from falling on my head onto concrete floors. In 2007 I had a stroke due to complicated migraine. I also lived in the woods of northern New England as an 18 to 22 year old, and many of my symptoms are consistent with the controversial diagnosis of chronic Lyme disease. It is in no way surprising that I live with chronic fatigue and inflammation, joint and muscle pain, multiple food sensitivities that make eating a balanced diet an incredibly intricate undertaking, and severe environmental illness that makes most public spaces, including buses, stores, libraries, theaters and the offices of doctors and therapists inaccessible to me.

Unfortunately, our health care system is not set up to recognize, research or heal the emerging chronic illnesses, that reckless industrial development and disregard for ecological consequences have made epidemic. The constellation of ills that impact the immune, neurological and endocrine systems, with their fluctuating symptoms and multiple causes, don't respond well to a medical model designed to deal with infectious diseases, where it's assumed that "real" illnesses have consistent symptoms and single causes.

In spite of the fact that I was raised middle class, am highly educated, and am an internationally known author whose writing is widely taught in universities, I have lived my adult life in poverty, unable to consistently hold a job, and unable to afford adequate medical care, the most effective of which is offered by integrative medicine doctors not covered by insurance. Over the decades, my health has deteriorated, and now, at 59, I am once again financially dependent on a now aged parent.

When this current disaster struck, I send out an appeal for help, and the most remarkable thing happened. I got it. Donations flowed in from friends, yes, but mostly from readers, from people familiar with the writing that, in spite of everything that conspired to stop me, I have continued to create. I received enough money to cover my attendant care for several months. I feel incredibly proud that my work has moved so many people to the point that they want to support my survival with cash, and incredibly grateful.

So when the money ran out once more, I thought I would pull together a chapbook of unpublished works, something to offer as a premium to persuade already generous donors to donate again. But when I started rummaging around in my files, I discovered that I had a whole book's worth of writing about bodies, from a prose poem about the 19th century politics of brown women's sexuality to the soundtrack to a dance I choreographed and performed about my stroke, from a praise song for my wheelchair to an essay on healing justice. I had my blogs from the ten weeks I spent receiving medical care in Cuba, and more recent blogs on the environmental causes of epilepsy, the health care potential of epigenetics and the everyday experience of being sick..

Kindling was an act of desperation, created out of an urgent need to raise some money. It is also evidence of the resilience that speaking one's truth can bring to the most dire of circumstances. Because, in spite of pain and poverty, sickness and fear, sexual violence and medical abuses, I have continued to speak my truth, and it has saved me. May my truth stand beside yours, and do its part in the task of saving us all.

You can follow my blog at:

www.auroralevinsmorales.com.

You can also make direct donations to support my ongoing survival at:

www.auroralevinsmorales.com/donate.html

MOUNTAIN

MOVING DAY

Mountain Moving Day:

*A Talk Given Via Skype at the Gloria Anzaldúa Conference
in San Antonio, Texas, 2010*

Dear Gloria—

Well, here it is el Día de las Muertas again and I've come to sit with you awhile. The living are busy trying to excavate your soul, writing all kinds of papers about the meaning of your life, spinning analyses from your words, arguing about the true significance of when you said this or that, digging up quotes to prove that you do or don't posthumously support hundreds of positions on thousands of issues. It's the usual mix of thoughtful insight and the absolute nonsense people invent when they're forced to churn out theory in order to keep their jobs in the middle of a depression. Some of them, I'm sorry to say, have even canonized you! I know. It's a hell of a thing to do to a flawed human being just because she had some great ideas and a strong writing hand and told her own truths. People are desperate for guides, so they remake us into oracles, and miss half the lessons our lives could offer them.

The questions on this particular table are about why you refused to identify as a disabled woman, and what illness and pain have to do with what you called the Coatlicue state, that well-mapped region of chaotic breakdown leading to revelation.

That question about how people identify, which battles we take on and how and when and with whom, gets so loaded with judgment, with accusations of having let down the team, with diagnoses of self-betrayal by those who made different choices. We choose which ground to fight on for such a mix of reasons: what feels urgent, what feels hopeful, whether we have a good band of fighters to stand with, how much of ourselves we can bring to each struggle. I spent years reading the lives of early 20th century Jewish feminists, trying to decipher what led them to fight on the terrains of gender, class and Jewishness in varying combinations. So much depends on solidarity.

In the late 70s and early eighties there was no place for me to stand as a bisexual woman. The fluidity of "queer" did not yet exist, and the lines of sexual identity were rigidly drawn. The oppression was bitterly painful, between the toxicity of heterosexism on one side and the often brutal rejection by lesbians on the other, cutting me out of the places I most longed to be. But there was not yet a critical mass of people I could fight beside to claim my place.

Most of the rooms I entered in those years were impossible to bring my whole self to, for many different reasons. But some of those silencings, those barriers, were being thought about and struggled over by many, many people, and we took it on together. So I fought about racism and then about anti-Semitism, and the battles were difficult and complex, (as a Jew of color, they still are,) but there was often critical mass. I had enough people who shared enough ground that I could fight for myself and others, win some battles, and not be demolished.

For you to shout out to the world, "Hey, not only am I a dark skinned working class Tejana lesbian, but I'm disabled, too!," to draw attention to yet another way you were oppressed, and for this to do you good, you would have needed a strong, vocal, politically sophisticated, disability justice movement led by queer working class women and trans people of color who understood your life, and it wasn't there yet. You would have needed people who saw that all the ways our bodies are made wrong, held responsible for our own mistreatment, blamed for showing the impact of oppression, all the ways our nature is called defective, are connected, rooted in the same terrible notions about what is of value. Who would have understood to the core your reasons for brewing all those herbal teas, knowing it's dangerous to enter the doors of the medical-industrial complex, and that there are things we need in there.

If you were here now, maybe what we've been constructing these last few years would be enough, would look to you like a place to rest, to be known. Oye, comadre, sometimes history leaves us stranded, waiting for a train that's still being built, five or ten years up the tracks. Have some pan dulce. Can't touch it myself, what with the diabetes and the gluten allergy, but the dead can eat whatever they want.

What I'm really interested in is that state you named after your ancestral goddess, the Coatlicue state, in which a shattering lets in light. Of course being Boricua not Mexica I call it the Guabancex and Oyá state, after the storm goddesses, the deities of creative destruction, of my Taino and West African ancestors. The landscape of my homeland is regularly uprooted by hurricanes, those wild, whirling, spirals of wind and water spreading out vast arms out to pluck trees and houses and lives from solid land, drive bits of metal right through tree trunks and take giant bites out of cement.

In the structure of a hurricane, the strongest, deadliest winds are closest to the core, but the core itself is clear, calm, full of light. Illness has been one long hurricane season for me, chunks of cement and metal roofing flying through the air, big trees made into heaps of splinters and shredded roots. What takes me to the core, to the place of new insight is listening with all my being to the voice of my own flesh, which is often an unbearable task. What lets me bear it is political, is a deep, ecological sense of the web in which my flesh is caught, where the profound isolation of chronic illness forces me to extend my awareness beyond individual suffering, beyond the chronic pain of my muscles and joints, the endless exhaustion, the mind-bending build up of toxins where nausea and nightmare meet, dragging me from my bed at three am to lift cups of bitter tinctures my lips with cramping hands, and leach the poison from my own liver.

In the steepest pitch, the darkest hour, in the ring of deadly wind, the only salvation is to expand, to embrace every revelation of my struggling cells, to resist the impulse to flee, and hold in my awareness both things: the planetary web of life force of which I am part, and the cruel machinery that assaults us: how greed strips and poisons landscapes and immune systems with equal disregard, how contempt for women, and the vastly profitable medical-industrial complex conspire to write off as hysterical hundreds of thousands of us bearing witness through decades in bed, while we're told all we need is a change of attitude.

To think, for example, not just about the side effects of anti-seizure drugs, or the need for stable sleep, but also society's hatred of unruly bodies, the frequent killing of epileptics by cops, and those 20th century eugenicists who built "colonies" to protect society from our bad seed, yes, the same people who sterilized 37% of all Puerto Rican women of child-bearing age, the same people who traveled to Nazi Germany to lecture about building a master race.

When my body feels as if it's tearing itself apart, when I'm in the nightmare condition, shaking and nauseated, my vision full of flashing lights, my legs too weak to stand, the only path out is deeper. Did you hear that Mami has cancer in the marrows of her bones? For her the key to peace is acceptance and a mind fixed on the present, but for me the material roots of my illness and hers are essential, medicinal, and rage clarifies things for me. I need to map it, and not just for myself. Our bodies, the bodies of two Caribbean women who were born and grew up in the 20th century, amidst war and industry and political repression, hold political truths about the world we live in, about damage and resistance, about truth telling and healing, and so did yours, with its infant bleeding and rocketing glucose.

There are days when I pretend I have no body, not to enter the windstorm of physical, spiritual, emotional and political pain that waits there. Sometimes clarity is intolerable. If I write about our bodies I will be writing about the "chemical revolution" that began by retooling leftover weapons into peacetime product, and has saturated our environment with 100,000 new molecules, which, in a reckless euphoria of avarice, we were all blithely assured would bring better living to all. If I write about our bodies I am writing about the land and what has been done to it. I am writing about unbreathable cities and abandoned coffee farms and tainted water, about starvation and death by thirst deliberately built into business plans. I am writing about the agricultural choices forced on people whose economic lives are ruled from afar, of shade trees clear cut for slightly higher production, leaving a wake of cancer and erosion, of massive advertising campaigns to persuade Puerto Rican women that canned vegetables and Tang are more "civilized" than fresh calabaza and orange juice, about what crossing the border does to the Mexicana pancreas.

And going in, going deeper, allowing the pain, there is the moment when I come clear: this isn't just a tale of damage. It's also a chart of where we need to go. The transformation of the planet into a sustaining and sustainable eco-social system moves along pathways we can't entirely see, but with their hungers and injuries and amazing capacity for renewal, our bodies have both a great store of critical information, and something like night vision. These three bodies I am writing about, my mother's, my own and yours, are not "statistically significant" but we have other significance. We are not representative, but we are extremely relevant.

The mountain moving day is coming. DDT on my father's work clothing entered the fatty tissue of my toddler body and is still there. Parathion sprayed in our home against disease-carrying mosquitoes ignites the nerve pathways in my brain. Sexual violence has impaired my digestion and increased the excitability of my neurons. *I say so yet others doubt it.* Formaldehyde leaking from new carpets and particleboard in the place we moved to when I was pregnant has left tracks of hysteria throughout my immune system. *Only a while the mountain sleeps. In the past all mountains moved in fire.* All over the world women sick in bed are thinking about these things. Those of us with electricity and computers and literacy write to each other. Susan in Santa Fe and Maria in Cayey and Beverly on Vashon Island and Julie in Arizona and Lisa in Washington, DC and Naomi in New York City. All over the world people whose bodies tremble and mutate, whose lungs labor, who sweat and cramp and can't remember what they were saying, are making connections. *Yet you may not believe it.*

Gloria if you were here now, among us, with your endlessly bleeding womb and glucose making tidal waves in your blood, you would not be silent about this, because you would not be alone. I think if we called on you to bring the story of your body to this circle, you would come.

There is no neutral body from which our bodies deviate. Society has written deep into each strand of tissue of every living person on earth. What it writes into the heart muscles of five star generals is distinct from what it writes in the pancreatic tissue and intestinal tracts of Black single mothers in Detroit, of Mexicana migrants in Fresno, but no body stands outside the consequences of injustice and inequality. *O man, this alone believe.*

These words are the lyrics to a creative collaboration across time between late 19th and early 20th century Japanese feminist poet Yasano Akiko and Naomi Weisstein, born in 1939, feminist psychologist, neuroscientist and founder of the Chicago Women's Liberation Rock Band, and it was the soundtrack to my awakening as a young feminist in Chicago in the late 1960s and early 1970s. I saw it silkscreened onto posters by members of the Chicago Women's Graphics Collective with whom I lived after I dropped out of high school in 1970. *All sleeping women now awake and move.*

All women whose muscles ache with permanent inflammation, all women who find lumps, all women whose babies miscarry one after another, whose life expectancy is stunted by malnutrition, who, because of industrial farming and "free trade" no longer own plots of land to grow food, who work in dangerous factories or sell sex in urban slums. My body and your bodies make a map we can follow.

We are connected to every jobless reservation and scarred, stripped tract of rainforest, every factory takeover and vacant lot community garden, every malaria death and clean water project, every paramilitary gang and people's constituent assembly. Our bodies are in the mix of everything we call political.

What our bodies, my mother's and yours and mine, require in order to thrive, is what the world requires. If there is a map to get there, it can be found in the atlas of our skin and bone and blood, in the tracks of neurotransmitters and antibodies. We need nourishment, equilibrium, water, connection, justice. When I write about cancer and exhaustion and irritable bowels in the context of the treeless slopes of my homeland, of market driven famine, of xenoestrogens and the possible extinction of bees, I am tracing that map with my fingertips, walking into the heart of the storm that shakes my body and occupies the world. As the rising temperature of the planet births bigger and more violent hurricanes from the tepid seas, I am watching the needle of my anger swing across its arc, locating meridians, looking for the magnetic pulse points of change. When I can hold the truth of my flesh as one protesting voice in a multitude, a witness and opponent to what greed has wrought, awareness becomes bearable, and I rejoice in the clarity that illness has given me. As my aching body and the storm-wracked body of the world tumble and spin around me, I enter the clear eye at the heart of all this wild uprooting, the place our sick bodies have brought us to, where light breaks through, and we can see the pattern in the broken forests and swollen waters and aching flesh—the still and shattered place where transformation begins.

Bombazo

*(Bomba is a traditional Afro-Puerto Rican music and
dance form now experiencing a major revival. This piece
was written for a conference on women in bomba.)*

Ponce, 1881. Controlling women's bodies is the key to the
gate, the beams under the floor, the roof on the house of race
and inheritance, and dark women's bodies are the fence posts
on the boundaries of power. On one side of the fence there is
honor and virtue, which means white women who only give
it up for the one man they have a contract with, before family,
God and law, and the white men who hold the deeds to them.
On that side of the line, decent isn't about how you treat people,
it's about whose fingers go where. Controlled women make
everyone respectable.

But to have decent, honorable, white, you have to have indecent,
scandalous, Black—something to be the opposite of. To keep
a tight hold on White in a Caribbean nation full of mestizaje,
where it doesn't take but a minute to mix the red wine blood of a
straying Mallorquina or a pale criolla kept out of the sun just to
be safe, with the burnt sugar amber fire of a seventh generation
barrio Mandinka, or put green eyes from Galicia on the brown
baby of la negra Malén, you can't just rely on the color of skin.
People have to act white; there has to be a whole list of white
ways to act, which means you have to have an opposite list of
Black ways to act and not act that way.

High up on the list of how a woman can act white is to never walk
alone, talk loud, or go out without a chaperone, to dance with

decorum and keep her skirt down and her shirtwaist buttoned. The dark people who get rewarded for acting white are mostly men, and no matter what they look like, most poor women in the cities and coastal towns act Black. They talk back, they don't obey, they walk all over the place, and what they dance is not European. A woman who "acts Black" is an uppity woman and an uppity woman is a loose woman, immoral, scandalous, without shame, because every slaveholder's grandson knows that dark women are just like that. You could be the best behaved dark skinned girl in the barrio, but no white man will believe it. You could be a moon white jíbara girl just down from the hills, but if you go to the bomba dance you just got five shades darker. Let me hear you say *Bomba!*

White men loyally supporting the power of the Spanish Crown, white men daringly and eloquently calling for autonomy, mulato artisans arguing for their own citizenship in these changing times, sober working men of all colors, and ardent white feminists demanding to go to school all agree: unruly scandalous disrespectful streetwalking bomba dancing out of control dark skinned women who don't know their place have got to be dealt with for civilization to march into the coming century. Time to start rounding up the women. *Bomba!*

Its been twenty years since abolition, and now dark women fill the streets of Ponce, working for themselves. Market women, laundresses, seamstresses, the coins they earn go into their own pockets. They rent houses together. They talk loudly in the streets.

And if wrongful power still stinks up the air they breathe, these days they can breathe a whole lot more of it. At night the hardworking women of Ponce pool their money and hire coaches. They go in laughing groups to taverns where they drink and flirt. They sing and strut and call out teasing verses, clap their hands and then they all shout *Bomba!*

1894. A woman you can't control is a prostitute. No proof needed. If you are a suspect you have to register. Things for which you can become a suspect: Talking back to a shopkeeper. Being outdoors at night. Having a man in your house. Unseemly dancing. Most of the women accused of prostitution are dark. You know why.

OK, lets' get something straight right now. It was a time of ruined crops and failing markets, of women drifting into the towns from countrysides of hunger, when poor folks lived in piles of sticks and mud and palm thatch that rotted in the rains, and every mouthful counted, every loaf of bread, every half pound of beans. The ones who had work, who had a pretty dress and ate enough, and whose children had something to wear, all knew how much worse it could get, so don't get all shocked.

Of course women traded sex for food. We always have. Sex for food, sex for shelter, sex for clothing against the cold, and even in Ponce, when it's raining and it's nighttime and your walls are made of sticks, it gets cold. The ladies did it for life and the women of the barrios temped, and mostly it was just one of the dozen things they did to hold things together and feed their kids: wash the señora's sheets, make dulce de coco to sell in the plaza, sew dresses, hem pants, and lie down for men.

Sometimes there was a man with a bit of money, a blanquito or a well paid craftsman who wanted a mistress, and that was better than marrying because there was not even the dream of divorce, and he might set her up in a house, pay the bills for a while, give her something for the children they made and she raised. So I'm not saying that some of the women who got hauled in and humiliated, pass-booked and segregated didn't trade bootie for cash. If you think it's indecent, so's making toxic sneakers for pennies in a sweatshop, stitching cheap t shirts in a high death rate maquiladora, or having to serve styrofoam wrapped carcinogenic fast food to children for minimum wage. Talk about obscene. Everybody shout *Bomba!*

Meanwhile back in Ponce it's 1895. Arrests are up and more and more of the arrested end up in jail. Anything a woman does that draws attention to herself is grounds for suspicion: walking by herself, dancing with a registered woman, leaving her parents' house after dark. Dancing in an African way. Any man can denounce a woman as having a venereal disease and that's that. Rejected lovers, angry boyfriends, resentful neighbors, people with grudges—anyone can accuse her and there is no trial. Her name goes on a list and now she has to carry a passbook. Maybe she's forced to move to a different part of town, away from the big houses.

The people with power are obsessed with the idea that she is infectious, that something about her will sneak into their houses and destroy the foundations of their lives. It isn't really VD but they say it's VD. So every two weeks registered women have to come to the station and have a public pelvic exam. Yes, you heard me right. The public hygiene doctors make them lie down on a table, in front of the policemen and any spectators who happen to have wandered by, spread their legs and have unsterilized metal instruments shoved into their bodies while all these men stand around and watch. If it turns out some guy did give them syphilis or gonorrhea they lock them up in a special hospital with spiked fences, bars on the windows, rotten food and violent guards, and since hospitals are not jails, they don't have to set any date for release. Don't think the poor women of Ponce surrendered. They forged passbooks, denounced men who didn't pay what they promised, shouted insults at the guards from the windows of the hospital, made ropes out of sheets and climbed out, and every chance they got, they danced. *Bomba!*

Now the authorities start cracking down on bomba dancing, which they call *bailes de prostitutas,* shutting them down every chance they get, because let me tell you, if the men's hands rising and falling on the taut heads of the drums, surrendering to no one, raising up a beat full of the spirits of slave revolts, reminding them of Cuba's Black general Maceo who right that moment is riding across sugar fields leading a multitude of dark men with machetes in hand, if the flying hands of the men scare them—it's the women's hips that terrify them into a cold sweat panic, those white skirts hiked up to show ankles, legs, even a glimpse of thighs that belong to no one, unlicensed willful women, imitating hens in heat, shaking their backsides at the drummers, because if women like this belong to nobody, if no one can make them fold their hands in their laps, if they can be possessed of their own selves like that, then anything can happen, and maybe some people think it's the drummers who matter most, but it's the uncontrolled fire of brown women's bodies that shakes the ground beneath the feet of church and state.

Transfusion

for Marcie Rendon

this is for the donors of blood, the ones

who transfuse the courage of their hearts

into the faltering world

who tax the endurance of their bones

and farm their own marrow

for the sake of what everyone needs,

until it cries out for a season of fallows-

but if the if red cells fail,

who will carry this oxygen on their backs

so that the People continue to breathe?

this is to say that this morning, I will breathe words

mouth to mouth, into the lungs of the suffocating,

that I have no hands or feet or back to offer, but today

I will breathe for as many as I can

and you

lie still

let the earthworms make soil

out of dead leaves and

broken limbs,

turn our beloved dead into rich dark cores of red

in the ivory hollows of your legs, ribs, shoulders.

let new blood well up

from the great aquifers of the earth,

and rise into your limbs, eyes, fingertips

like the green, sweet sap

no one can imagine in midwinter.

Be still. Make blood.

I will breathe.

Take-Back

Take Back the Night, Bellingham, Washington, April, 2001

Take back the night of Janet walking to her car after a movie, humming to herself, stopping to pull out her keys, thrown against the side of the car, dragged down, filthy rag over her face, someone muttering, hissing threats in her ear, cold metal on her cheek says its a knife, too scared to think, raped right there on the gravel of the parking lot, and when he jumps up and takes off down the alley, rolls over and vomits under her car, goes home, stands in the shower for hours trying to wash it away. Take back all the nights since then that she doesn't leave the house, won't go places alone, can't stand her girlfriend's touch, sits shaking in the car, parks only on busy streets, has the campus escort service walk her from her evening class to the main lot, jumps at the sound of anyone behind her anywhere. Those streets she used to walk alone on summer nights, that man whose face she never saw took them away from her. She takes self defense classes, reads strategies, carries a whistle, does all the powerful things to protect herself, knows how to defend herself and nevertheless can't forget, knows with all her vigilant senses that at a moment's notice she could once again be prey.

Take back Donna's nights, knowing from the set of his shoulders it's one of those times, breathless chatter putting the food on the table trying to head him off but no surprise when he throws the dinner she made him at the wall and makes her clean it up, asks her what the hell good she is, smacks the side of her head so hard her ears ring, tells her to quit crying it's her own damn fault, sorry, sorry but you made me so mad, you really shouldn't do that, sorry baby sorry kissing the bruises while she fights down nausea, don't leave me, don't you even try to leave me, you know we belong together and I'd kill you sooner than let you go, kill you, while she tries to imagine what it would be like to hear the front door open and not be afraid, to eat what she wants whenever she wants and go out and come in with no-one to answer to, wondering where there might be a doorway out of here between pity, shame and terror, between wishing him different, and wanting him dead.

Take back Patty's nights as she listens for footsteps in the hall that will hesitate outside her door, the creak of the hinge, the rustling of his pants as he walks slowly to her bedside where she's pretending to be asleep, the tug of the sheets as he pulls them back, and pulls up her nightie and begins to touch her, the little whistle in his breath after a while, the jerking movements, the sticky places, her eyes squeezed tight to not believe in what is happening, the stories she tells herself to make it a fairy tale of monsters that vanish or turn into stone. Take back the nights she lies awake doing math puzzles calculating how many seconds it will be until she's old enough to drive a car and drive all the way away from here, two hundred sixty eight million seven hundred and seventeen thousand six hundred and fifty-six seconds, fifty-five, fifty-four, fifty-three.

Take back the night for Johnetta listening to the echoes of night sticks and metal doors slamming shut, down long corridors of anguish rage loneliness times 800 women simmering behind bars, as she tries to conjure up the smell of her youngest baby's skin, milk and sweat sweet, her memory fighting for control of her senses, against the acrid prison laundry bleach and fear stench of her sheets, nine years, and only eleven months down still eight years and one month to go. Her baby will be half grown before she gets out of here caught with a thimbleful of coke but one thing adds to another and it's a strike, another dark woman working for pennies and punishment, trapped by slavers, trying to stay alive and sane while someone else listens to her children breathe in their sleep and hears their stories and watches them outgrow their shoes.

Take back Tina's night, six months ago on a Saturday she and her brother Freddy and a couple a friends kickin' it, walking down the street eleven o clock just laughing, talking, headed home when three squad cars screech in around them, surround them, and Angela and Rafi take off, but one a them has a billy club pressed tight against Pancho's throat, and Freddy says no man, leave him alone you're choking him as Pancho gags and coughs, then two a them jump Freddy, throw him to the ground, shove his face into the concrete, and Tina screams while another one twists her arms behind her back demanding to know what gang are you in, damn Mexicans even though she and Freddy are from Honduras and Pancho is Salvadoran. And then when Freddy turns his head, trying desperately to breathe, she sees it over and over now, the two who have him down start kicking him, clubbing him in a rage of hatred like they can't stand to see anybody brown alive and laughing, and she keeps screaming leave him alone, he didn't do nothin', somebody help us, while they drag Tina back and shove her in a squad car with Pancho and take them to the station. It's many hours later before her mother manages to bail her out and by that time Freddy is cold, no more laughing, and now Tina walks down the street like a volcano ready to vomit fire.

Take back their nights and give the streets to Janet and Tina. Let Janet and Tina decide how to protect the laughing, the humming, the summer night walking of all of us and give them the entire budget of the Los Angeles Police Department to do it with. Take back their nights and appoint Johnetta and Patty and Donna to write and carry out the family law that will celebrate every kind of loving and intervene against every kind of abuse, and reassign the entire personnel of the US Navy to help them do the job.

Go on and take back the corner by the porn shop, and the racks of splay-legged women wrapped in plastic, and make it into a safe sex teen education center. But take back also the oak paneled room on some twentieth floor in another city where all those five dollar rentals from videos that twist and poison the loneliness of sad and frightened men into brief and violent illusions of power and connection, pile up in corporate accounts, millions upon millions for marketing the fantasies of doing things to our bodies as a quick fix for pain. Turn the mansions of pornography's shareholders into rehab centers and art schools, give the oak paneled room to the ministry of joyous sex and set the board members to sweeping streets.

Take back all these nights in which we have been hunted, but take back also the afternoons of Micheline, working in the Megatex factory in Port Au Prince, Haiti for 27¢ an hour, which means she can eat or pay rent on a one room shack she shares with three younger siblings but not both, sewing Winnie the Pooh children's wear for Disney, Tigger fleece jackets that will sell, each one, for enough to support them all for weeks, so her little sister fucks middle aged men in the cemetery for a dollar a time to buy rice. Take back her afternoons from the violence wielded in distant board rooms, those contracts of global trade whose blows land in her life as brutally as the batterer's fist, and give her books and a living wage and the right to decide how to spend Disney CEO Michael Eisner's 9.9 million dollar bonus and his 565 million in stock options and his yearly salary of 750,000 to make Haiti a place people will no longer risk drowning to escape, a place where fourteen year olds eat rice anytime they're hungry, to find every single Haitian exile and invite all of them, joyously noisy in the brim-full airplanes of return, to come home.

Take back the afternoon of an anonymous woman testifying in secret in Guinea about the peaceful demonstration to release an opposition leader, how at two in the afternoon she was arrested, given forty lashes and then raped over and over again until she lost all sense, she says, of where she was. Take back the afternoon of Jeanette arrested in Burundi for collaborating with Hutu rebels because she is Hutu and was walking down a road carrying food, and Valérie, Elaine, Constance, Fitina and Sabine, all Hutu, all arrested, tortured, held year after year without trial. Take back the afternoon of Victoriana and Francisca of Guerrero, Mexico who went into the fields to find Victoriana's ten year old grandson and Francisca's young brother-in-law because they had not returned from harvesting crops the day before, and who stumbled into a military camp where they were thrown to the ground, stripped and raped repeatedly by the soldiers of their own government, and who found out two weeks later that by the time this was done to them, the man and boy they loved had already been taken by these soldiers and killed. Take back the afternoon of a thirteen year old street girl arrested for petty theft and an 18 year old woman picked up for vagrancy both raped by the Manila police, whom no-one will denounce because if you do, they get even, and no-one does anything anyway, the judge shrugging, saying obviously the child was no virgin. Dispossess the governments that rape, torture and kill as routine procedures of power, that terrorize and bribe the boys they draft to numbly enact their will. Make these women and girls the peacekeepers and judges of the planet. Give them the treasuries of nations and the street children and market women of the world for their staff, and let them occupy the offices of the World Bank and have authority to settle all disputes and let the men with guns come before them for mercy.

Take back the afternoon of Kajal, twenty four years old and living in Iraqi Kurdestan, detained by six members of her husband's family and accused of adultery, and although pregnant, tortured and mutilated by them, the tip of her nose cut off while her husband's kin told her that as soon as her child was born she would be killed to protect their honor. Take back the afternoon she went from the hospital into hiding, moving from place to place for months until she escaped the country, learning her attackers were questioned and immediately released since the authorities sympathized with them, agreed that the honor of men is soiled when a woman in their family has any contact with any other man, when a woman is raped, when a woman refuses to marry the man they choose for her—and such soiling can only be cleansed with murder. Take back Kajal's afternoon of torment and praise her courage in the public square, and then set her to teaching honor to the children of her country and let her make love with whoever she wants by the light of day, unafraid, in a room of her own.

Take back the afternoons of Nahdrah and Sima, Mina and Nafisa living under the Taliban which made it a capital crime to walk anywhere without a male relative, or be seen by any man not in the family, even to a quarter inch of ankle. Take back the afternoons they spent sitting at home behind windows painted over to hide them, since the regime outlawed work and education for Afghani women and Dr. Mina could not practice medicine, Nafisa could not study geography, Sima learned arithmetic from a textbook hidden underneath the floor, Nahdrah still mourns her sister beaten to death for accidentally touching a man when she stumbled. Take back their days and from now on and for the next twelve hundred years, let them be the voices of spiritual wisdom that tell humanity how the righteous must conduct themselves in this world, with the joyous assent of all people.

Take back the afternoon of Ana Carmen sitting in the waiting room of the public hospital in Ponce, Puerto Rico for the doctor who doesn't bother, half the time, to show up from his private practice across town, even though she had to come two hours over mountain roads, her son taking off time from work to bring her so they can give her something for the pain that wakes her all night where the cancer is chewing through the bones of her legs and hips and back. She and her husband never spread the pesticides on their own crops, even though the extension agents won't give them seeds or tools if they refuse, but their neighbors did, and the poisons have seeped into the drinking water, contaminated the garden, coated their skins while they bathed, for over thirty years. The green revolution stripped the hills of trees and killed the birds and now it is stripping the flesh off her bones and making her bones crumble. Take back these waiting room afternoons smelling of antiseptic soap and sweat, and give her back her years and the forests and the lizard cuckoos that used to call in the valleys before the rain and give her the twenty year worldwide profits of Monsanto to plant slopes and renew immune systems and give seeds to the sowers of seed everywhere. Put Ana Carmen and the Palestinian villager whose olive trees were uprooted by tanks and the Indian rice farmer coerced into buying sterile seed, in charge of global food and farming, and give them the US, British and Israeli military budgets to do it with.

And now listen: the day will come when we will also take back the mornings and when it does, it will be more than freedom to walk home without attack. It will be waking to a world where attack is inconceivable. When we take back the mornings, the assaults of poverty will be an ancient obscenity our grandchildren study but cannot comprehend, staring at pages that recount how people starved to death while a handful squandered their lives in pursuit of luxuries, how corporations wrote our deaths from cancer into their development plans, how those wars in which soldiers raped women into unconsciousness were fought for mere possessions. When we take back the mornings, we will wake each day into a world where rape is so taboo that no boy will grow up thinking of it except with horror, where those afflicted with the greed to have more than everyone else are sent to detox clinics to break their addiction to wealth, where universities are filled with the children of the women who used to clean them, and classes are taught in the languages of the formerly dispossessed, in Mohawk and Quechua and Ohlone.

Right now, everywhere on this planet, women are turning the world toward morning, inch by inch, by hand. Women are slipping under fences tonight in Vieques, Puerto Rico, to put their bodies in the way of the US Navy's practice bombs. Women are smuggling girls out of Somalia and Burma to save them from mutilation and sexual slavery. Women are publishing truths on hand printed sheets of paper, testifying on the internet, linking arms across roads, raising money, training each other, vowing to uproot not only rape but the reasons for rape, to stop not only the soldiers but the trainers and employers of soldiers, not only one violation but all violations.

Walk out tonight into the streets with all of their steps beside yours. Feel the ground tremble. Walk out tonight chanting and hear the voices of women in Colombia, Thailand, Araucaria, Nigeria, Albania, Brazil, Ireland, Iraq, Diné. Lean forward, feet on the ground, and push. We are turning the world out of prehistory into that morning that will be ours, when everyone on earth will wake up unafraid.

Kindling

When I was a child the world was full of unusual things, astonishing realities. Just the thought that we were part of a galaxy which was one of millions, a speck of life in a vast expanse of space, made me shiver and sometimes kept me up at night. As a child you are both shocked by reality and take for granted that it's strange. That caterpillars wind themselves up in silk thread, dissolve their own bodies and remake themselves into butterflies. That blood races around inside our bodies. That people organize wars. Or insert parts of their bodies into other people's bodies and this results in new people. My brother and I thought that as we moved through the world, we left energy trails behind us and that at the end of life, it would be like letting go of one end of a stretched rubber band—-we'd go flying backwards along the path we'd traveled, only a lot faster— which is why we took care not to tangle our trails around lampposts our other people. We didn't want to get bruised.

So the fact that the flicker of sunlight through trees could make me feel like I was lifted out of my body, or those moments when time seems to slow to an excruciating crawl, my mouth was flooded with a taste like sucking on key chains, and I could move, didn't seem worth mentioning. Or those other flickers of consciousness, that feeling of having just arrived, just gotten back without any memory of leaving. The odd variations of my brain and body didn't seem out of place in a world with an aurora borealis or deep sea fish that dangled glow-in-the-dark blobs in front of their own mouths to catch prey.

At seventeen, when one of my close friends tells me she saw me jerking and making odd sounds, and remembering nothing about it later, it was in the context of a subculture of self-induced trances, ouija boards and spink, the imaginary drug with which we generated group hallucinations out of thin air.

So it was a shock to me, to wake up on a stair landing at 23 and be told by two hastily departing Spanish students, that I'd been convulsing. I had just spent the weekend in Yosemite. Four of us had backpacked across rock strewn valleys all the way to Young Lakes, a hefty hike with a heavy load at high altitude. It was cold, the ground was hard, I didn't sleep much and ate lightly. I rose at dawn and stepped, naked, into icy water as light sprang across sky and rock faces, and then we hiked back. I was out on three limbs I now know not to go out on: intense physical exertion, sleep deprivation and low blood sugar.

The next time was while I was in labor, and it changed my daughter's birth from the intended home water birth to an emergency c-section after many hours hooked up to machines in the county hospital. I was under tremendous pressure to take drugs that would have prevented me from breast feeding. But my first neurologist had said it was a low seizure threshold, not true epilepsy, and this seizure, too, had been triggered by extreme exertion, sleep deprivation and low blood sugar. So I refused.

Then, ten years later, I started having them more often. I was in a stressful relationship, and I was in peri-menopause. Between 1998 and 2008 I had thirteen tonic-clonic seizures — the kind where you fall down, thrash around, pee on yourself and bite your tongue to shreds. Seven of those were in a nine-month period after my divorce. I kept careful records, and I had been tracking my menstrual cycles since my teens, so when my naturopath asked about the timing of my seizures it was easy to see that they clustered around my period. I had catamenial epilepsy, closely tied to shifting hormone levels, and the changes leading up to menopause were creating a hormonal roller coaster with neurological earthquakes.

In 2005 I discovered the work of Donna Andrews and Joel Reiter. Reiter was the first neurologist I had consulted after the Yosemite-induced seizure. Donna Andrews was a woman who had had encephalitis, leading to ten seizures a day, and had learned to control them. She'd been seizure-free for 37 years and she and Dr. Reiter had a clinic where they were teaching other people to do what she did. So my family found the money and I spent five days in a hotel in Santa Rosa, California, learning to negotiate with my own brain. Based on her techniques, I was able to identify my personal danger zones—not just the common ones, but those specific to me: doing oral histories that filed my head with stories, but not having anywhere to put them; leaving Puerto Rico after a visit; too many bright colors all at once; intense excitement. I learned how to recognize and back away from the edge where my brain throws the reset switch. For me, that means sensory deprivation, visualizing balance between hemispheres, and using my own system of color-coded neurological states to calm my nervous system. Also passionflower tincture, and in emergencies, a half tablet of Ativan. Since my cycles stopped, I have not had any tonic-clonic seizures.

But this doesn't mean the book is closed. For one thing, my EEGs have always shown little bursts of spike and wave activity, tiny micro-seizures that don't spread, but are going on all the time. I still have those little slippages of time, a fraction of a second long, noticeable only as a miniscule blur. It means my brain is still vulnerable to grand mal seizures, though I haven't had one in three years. But beyond that, is the question of why any of this is happening at all. My doctors call it idiopathic epilepsy, meaning they don't know. But I have suspicions.

It is both shocking and unsurprising that in the thirty-three years since my first epilepsy diagnosis, not one neurologist has ever suggested environmental factors a possible cause, in spite of the fact that our environment is filled with neuro-disruptors designed to devastate the central nervous systems of insects. There are huge vested interests behind the pretense that profit driven science is safe, and that the massive amounts of toxic substances produced by that science have no significant negative impact on people or ecosystems. At every step, attempts to trace the connections between carcinogens and cancer are hampered, but at least people are aware carcinogens exist. No-one talks about epileptogens.

Perhaps one reason is that unlike carcinogens which produce cancer as an unintentional effect, these chemicals were developed specifically for the purpose of creating chaos in the nervous systems of living beings. Parathion is an organophosphate, one of the most dangerous of that highly dangerous class of chemicals. It is 30 times more toxic than DDT, and was used for mosquito eradication during my childhood. It was invented by German chemist Gerhard Schrader who worked for IG Farber. While researching organophosphate pesticides for agriculture, he and his team discovered tabun, sarin, and two other nerve gasses classified as weapons of mass destruction. Twenty-four IG Farber executives were tried for war crimes at Nuremberg (and later reinstated as directors of chemical companies.) The company set up a chemical plant next to Auschwitz that at its peak used 83,000 enslaved laborers, and one of its subsidiaries, Degesch, made Zyklon B, the substance used to murder people in gas chambers.

One way that scientists study epilepsy is to create it in laboratory animals. One way to do this is through a process called kindling. The animals are given repeated doses of electrical or chemical stimulation, below the level that would cause outright seizures on the spot, and over a period of weeks, this permanently lowers their seizure thresholds. Although there's no detectable damage to brain tissue, the kindled animals' brain function is altered. There are changes in the amygdala, hippocampus and cortex, and to receptors for the neurotransmitters glutamate and GABA, leading to a state of cellular hyper-excitability, signs of increased anxiety, depression and cognitive problems. One report notes that kindling is most effective when doses are several times a week rather than daily. More is not necessarily more damaging.

Two of the chemicals used to kindle the brains of rats in these studies are the pesticides dieldrin and lindane, both of which were used on my family's farm. As a fetus, infant and toddler, I was quite certainly exposed to repeated doses not big enough to make me convulse, but I see no reason to doubt that they charged through my young brain, resetting my thresholds, altering my neurochemistry, and turning me into a kindled child.

Healing Justice and the Potential for Community Based Science

These are series of speculations on what recent insights in a variety of areas of science could mean for a community based healing movement that includes amateur research infused with radical understandings of what we mean by health and environment, and high expectations for our own empowered capacity.

1

Epigenetics is what scientists call the discovery that events in our environments can change the outer skin of our genes, change the way in which they express themselves, turning them off and on depending on how our bodies read the conditions of life, and that those changes get passed on to our descendents. Dutch women who survived the famine of 1944 gave birth to low weight babies, as expected, but when their children grew up, they also had low weight babies. The story of hunger clung to their DNA and passed on the traits appropriate to a permanent famine. Combat veterans pass on the changes in their own bodies that come with the constant threat of sudden and violent death, and the DNA of their children born after the trauma wears a coat of camouflage, expressed in the symptoms of PTSD.

But if hunger and terror tattoo the skins of our genes with outdated survival manuals and a continuous stream of SOS signals, if the conscious acts of human beings to deprive each other of food and safety and life itself, mark us in inheritable ways, surely we can decide to mark ourselves, through an entirely different set of human acts, with messages of solace and solidarity, with a codex of healing.

2

Behavioral science has spent far too much time studying competition, aggression, and dominance, traits that are leading the planet to the brink of extinction. The study of solidarity will never get an NIH grant, but we who hope to avert disaster and cultivate a peaceful, just and sustainable future, must study it. When I am in Cuba, in spite of bad food and extremes of heat and humidity, in spite of tobacco smoke and perfume in the air, in spite of the daily frustrations of getting places and reaching people, my body thrives. It thrives because I am surrounded by people who actively wish me well, who go out of their way, except that mutual support is their way, to help me thrive. On top of the more communally oriented nature of Caribbean cultures, Cubans have consciously cultivated a sense of solidarity as the core value of their society. Immersion in that conscious culture did at least as much in my recovery from stroke, as the 40 hours a week I spent in physical therapy and other treatment. The work of healing justice must include the systematic study of the healing properties of solidarity, and develop ways to cultivate it even in the harsh conditions of a city like Oakland.

3

Neuroplasticity research has shown us that our brains are far more malleable, adaptive, *alive,* than the old mechanistic models could have dreamed of. Our brains can reroute nerve impulses through new pathways that are made with thought, can reassign whole sections to new functions, can restore what was thought to be broken or lost beyond recovery. We can visualize exercising, and create the benefits of exercise while lying in a bed with cast on. We can train the brain to recover from stroke and blows to the head. Using techniques from biofeedback, we can consciously alter the balance of brain wave frequencies and change aspects of depression, ADHD, the aftereffects of traumatic injury, by desiring dots on a screen to remain within a box. We can regain the use of stroke-weakened limbs, control body temperature, activate the visual cortexes of the blind using patterns of stimulation on their backs. The work of healing justice must include learning everything we can about conscious adaptation, about how to communicate directly with our brains, and then develop low tech practices for community based neurological restoration projects.

4

Type 2 diabetes is a disease of stress. The overworked pancreas begins to refuse its job, insulin receptors stop receiving, cells die and the flow of life-giving glucose starts surging wildly, endangering everything in its path: eyes, feet, heart, brain. Mexican migrants who cross the border, very quickly become many times more vulnerable to the disease. One obvious reason is dietary change, the exchange of beans and tortillas and fresh salsa for hamburgers on white bread and deep fried potatoes. But crossing the border also means entering a climate of hostility, uprooted from their place and people and language of origin. Stress releases hormones in the blood that call forth glucose from the body's stores. Continual stress exhausts the pancreas. Then we're told to cut out the foods that comfort us, exercise when we're bone weary from struggling, and do it as individual patients, on sheer willpower.

What if we told a different story about diabetes? What if we said the pancreas has gone on strike from loneliness, from homesickness, from uprootedness and isolation. What if we created healing cells made up of four or five diabetics whose job was to help restore each other's roots and cultivate group solidarity? What if they shared meals, cooked for each other twice a week, went on walks together, strategized about protecting their bodies from the stressors in their lives, cried and raged about what's been awful and unfair, practiced listening to their bodies' deepest hungers as a guide to diet? Tenderly chopped and cooked and seasoned what made them feel most at home in themselves. What if their story was not one of defective organs, unruly appetites and laziness? What if it was a story of homecoming?

5

For the last 27 years I've participated in the project of Re-Evaluation Counseling, (RC) a set of practices and theories about how we recover from being hurt, how emotional injury gets locked into us in the form of a stiffened set of false beliefs about reality, and how by bringing others with us to the inner place of wounding, we can make use of our bodies' natural methods of healing— crying, shaking, yawning, sweating, laughing—to release those hurts and see the world afresh. One of the many beauties of RC is the exquisite attention paid to the particular ways that historical hurts are stored within particular groups of people. Sorted by class, gender, ethnicity, nationality, sexuality, occupation, age, the accumulated expertise of RC provides a kind of field guide to the impact of oppression.

I now know how to recognize in myself the anxiety that appears as distrust of the competence of others, but is rooted in centuries of insecurity among my Ukrainian Jewish ancestors, handed down, I am sure, in both psychological and cultural patterns of feeling, thinking and acting, and as shifts in what my body responds to as threatening, etched by the light of torches and burning houses into the methyl layers of my genes.

I know about the distinctive traits that history tends to bundle up for people who share an experience: attempted genocide, migration, slavery, the suppression of one's language or religion. I know in minute detail the sheaf of maps that show how sexism penetrates the psyche and flesh. And using the techniques we've developed in more than half a century, I know how to release some of those burdens, revise some of the solidified untruths we take in like heavy metals, to reside in the slow moving, fatty tissues of our sense of self.

Healing justice will need to use this base of knowledge, these and other tools that allow us to re-evaluate, to re-interpret the meaning of what has happened to us, in a way that makes us free to act, free to change ourselves in every layer of our being, from what we believe about our intelligence to how the million islets of our pancreases respond to the call for sugar.

6

I do a workshop I call Bonework. In it, I ask participants to identify a key story of their family, one that is told over and over, part of the "who we are" of their immediate kinship. I have them turn it into a one sentence narrative: "My family all married lighter people in order to stop being Black and pass into white society," or "My grandfather was abandoned by his family in the middle of the night, as a boy of six, and never saw them again," or "When my father was called up before the House Un-American Activities Committee and walked out of the hearings, and called my mother to tell her, I jumped up and down and cheered."

Then I ask the storytellers to gather in small group and probe each other's stories, ask questions about who or what is missing, propose alternative interpretations, explore all the possibilities they can lay their hands on. We come back to the circle and everyone either restates the story or asks a question. The woman whose family married whiter says her ancestors did whatever they had to, even at tremendous cost, to see to it that their children survived. The grandchild of the abandoned boy learns that the time and place of the events hint at external violence tearing the family apart, that placing him where they did might have been for his best protection. And I reveal the constant fear that underlay the radical bravado of my childhood, the hysterical relief in those cheers.

We leave the workshop with new stories that open up different possibilities of self – trust. When I do this work with individuals, I look deeper, unearth the inherited social relations as well as beliefs, and invent acts of repair with weight in the present day world. A woman decides to set up a water trust to replace the rivers her grandfather dammed, which caused a famine in a specific band of Apache people. A singer must compose a song about the people her homesteading ancestors displaced.

7

My father had a massive heart attack at fifty-one. His own father died at forty-six, after five heart attacks had weakened his heart, so that it couldn't withstand the stress of infection from a spoiled milkshake. My grandfather's siblings also died of heart disease. This is a strong family history of a specific condition. I imagine the hearts of the Lehrer-Sonnensheim-Levinskies with branching blood vessels reaching out into causes that include poverty-stricken shtetls, pogroms, a diet heavy in butter and cheese and sour cream, the knowledge of a world left behind and destroyed, the Type A life of communist organizers in the 1930s.

So far, my heart shows no allegiance to that heritage, but I did inherit eight blocked paths, eight genetic variations in the P450 cytochrome enzymes that regulate liver function, eight incapacities to convert and carry away the toxins that come in from the outside, or are created within my body. One of the blockages prevents the efficient breakdown of dopamine, estrogen and norepinephrin. Another increases my risk of cancer from tobacco smoke, diesel fumes, burnt meat and pesticides. A third makes me vulnerable to alcoholism and depression, but protects me from schizophrenia.

A major sport among my Puerto Rican relatives is genetic speculation. My cheekbones, they all agree, are like the second daughter of the third brother. Do I tend to wake up cranky?

That's *morra,* and is inherited from the Moures, while bad tempers came into our family with Jose María Hernandez, a Spanish soldier stationed in San Juan in the 19th century, who married a Morales daughter and cursed us with the tendency to shout. They say that thyroid disease runs in the deeply inbred Morales clan, along with square heads and stick-out ears.

My great aunts are more concerned with character traits and recognizable signs of kinship than inherited vulnerability to the smoke of cigars, or an inability to clean up a spill of stress hormones.

But this is what interests me. If gene expression is vulnerable to intense experience, if we can both inherit and alter the stories by which our bodies function, if the tracks of some of these traits are clearly to be seen among the Díaz clan, others obviously Morales, Lehrer, or Sakhnin, then let's invent a psycho-social-genetic-cardio-endocrine storytelling practice, something that uses the shovel of memory and metaphor to dig around in the whole question of history and heredity, and see what we can jiggle loose. Between the genealogical gossip of my relatives and the wisdom of my flesh, maybe I can discover and retell a story, brought down, perhaps, from the hills above Naranjito where my Taino ancestors survived the attempted extermination of their people, that will reinterpret the experiences of my ancestors and alter the expression of those liver enzyme genes to handle adrenal stress hormones in a whole new way.

What if we incorporate the researching and retelling of our family stories into our medical practice? What if we use the release and re-evaluation tools of RC alongside this intimate excavation of family history and family myth, and create a psychosocial surgery where we operate on the past, and create new endocrine and neurological and psychological interpretations of the present?

STRICKEN

Night Vigil

I know what time the clock says it is, but my body is in some other galaxy where day and night are random stripes of dark and light, unrelated to waking and sleeping. The last time I fell asleep, it was eight in the morning after a long night of excruciating pain in my right sacro-ileac joint and a knot in my gut, in the spot called the ileocecal valve. It's an old pain, long familiar to me, but this has been the worst episode I can remember. Inflammation in my gut overflowing its bounds and sending sharp agony outward in spirals through my whole body.

When the valve between the small and large intestines is irritated and jams open, toxins from the bowel flood back into the area meant for processing food and I slip into another familiar terrible state, a nightmarish semi-consciousness of auto-intoxication, where I drift on the surface of sleep, but can't sink. Finally at eight, wary of the thresholds of epilepsy, I take Benedryl and Ativan and sleep for a few hours.

Tracing the tendrils and roots of this crisis back through weeks of gathering symptoms, I remember that I added several new supplements to my routine, wanting to boost my detox power. My liver is hampered by nine genetic defects. It's as if instead of loading the by products of eating onto fast trains to be hauled away, my body must fill hand baskets a spoonful at a time and carry them away on foot.

It's not that my liver can't move toxic sludge, but it can't go very fast. So I have to help out however I can. I don't burden my organs with fried foods, red meat or pesticides, and I take supplements to enhance my liver's abilities. Milk Thistle and Bupleurum, Fringe Tree and Bog Bean, and I just started taking liposomal glutathione, a recent breakthrough that allows fragile oral glutathione, essential to the chemical processes of the liver, to actually make it into my bloodstream. I've also added NAC and Alpha Lipoic Acid, precursors to let my body make even more glutathione. Maybe it was too much. (One of the experts on mercury chelation says alpha lipoic acid can be hazardous, releasing mercury into the bloodstream faster than it can be gotten rid of. Others say it's all good. I am a juggler of expert advice.)

About two weeks after adding all this stuff, my gut started to rumble and my stomach began hurting in the morning when I woke up, sharp stabbing pain right up in my actual stomach, which was hard and tender to the touch. Then I broke out in hives all over my back and my face and arms swelled up. It took five days of antihistamines for them to go away. While I was on them, my stomach felt better. When I stopped, it got worse. Soon I couldn't eat anything without instant retribution in pain and diarrhea. But is this a sign of too rapid detox, a new set of food intolerances, increased irritation from the added fiber of springtime vegetables, the kale and raspberry smoothies that flow from my brand new Vitamix?

Then, the long awaited visit to my Lyme doctor, and the startling news that I also have a rare genetic defect in my immune system, that my body's likely loaded with spirochetes, twirling their way through my brain like tiny roto-tillers, and that with the nine closed gateways of my liver, I am probably awash in neurotoxins, not to mention the leftover pesticides of my 1950s childhood on a tropical farm. With all that load of poisons and my slowed waste disposal, my body is in no condition to try killing the little buggers. My elimination systems are too swamped with old business. He decides to start me on Ketotifen, a drug that stops leaky mast cells from dribbling histamine all over my gut, making inflammation and eventually wearing holes through the lining.

I start slow, since the stuff knocks me out, and my slow liver means every dose needs to be fractioned. The pain in my stomach and gut is really bad and the first dose seems to calm it some. Second day, too. Third day the pain is back and I try adding a tiny bit more in the afternoon. I sleep for hours, having hit some tipping point in the drug's sedative effects. Fourth day, I'm sitting at the table when my back suddenly and dramatically shifts into extreme pain. I can't sit, can't rise from my seat without yelling, can't bend, can't find any position that doesn't hurt like hell. It feels like burning metal is piercing a spot halfway between my spin and my hip, and nothing will make it stop. At the same time, on the front, something has twisted my intestines into a small, tight knot just inside the curved ridge coming down from my hip bone. It's been like this for four days.

I want to be writing my book. I want to be finishing the design of my fabulous new match making site. I want to be planting the garden, writing to a political prisoner, finishing hemming my daughter's shirt, embroidering, applying for an arts residency. All I can do is roll around and moan and it feels like such a dreadful waste of time.

Between the pain, and the sole responsibility of shuffling and sorting and laying out the details of my experience, seeking a pattern I can believe in, that will guide me to reasonable courses of action, sleep is elusive. It's dark again. I know that at four a.m. the birds will begin singing in the trees outside these windows. In the maple out front, not the blossoming dogwood. The beginning of bird song is one of the few landmarks of the deep night. It's still early enough to call California without waking anybody up. If I slept now, it would be a good night's sleep. But I can feel the toxins crawling along my nerves, making my body restless, edgy, making my skin crawl. Sometimes I wonder if my cells glow in the dark. At the microscopic level, do the molecules of mercury and parathion and inflammatory substances shimmer and gleam?

I have been sitting too long in my ergonomic chair. The pain is starting to build again in my back, and my stomach has begun to burn. It's a long time before the birds will start dropping their liquid notes through the new-leafed branches. I think I'll try peppermint tea this time.

Burnt Light

Many years ago I was trained in Model Mugging, a powerful form of self-defense based on the physical advantages of female rather than male bodies. We practiced the moves over and over until they were ingrained, learned at the level of nerve and muscle. Our teachers wanted our bodies to go on automatic if the need arose. And that does seem to be how it works. We were told a story about a woman who was attacked at a subway station, eight years after she graduated from the training. She didn't even remember the name of the course, but her body flew into action and carried out its moves without her. She has no recollection of what she did to her attacker. She had to deduce it from the hospital reports of the damage done.

I can't tell you what my body does when it has a grand mal, tonic-clonic seizure. My nervous system decides it's had enough and throws a switch and I go down. There's a lightning storm that I never see. I wake up in the landscape of its aftermath, in a field of debris, and trace its path by the damage done. I wake up incoherent, stumbling after words, language shredded and scattered, my tongue bloody, my pants drenched in urine. Burnt light, is what I say this time. Over and over, whispering to myself. Burnt light.

I wake up in the middle of a sentence, half an hour into a conversation, the first part of which is hidden from me. This time it's my niece telling me "She died." She died?! "When," I ask. "Of what? Was I there?" Because it seems I was asking for my mother. I often wake up asking for someone who is missing, so I must be aware, somewhere inside me, of a gap. Or else I was just with her. I ask if I still live on California Street, trying to figure out which chapter of my life I'm in right now. It could be any one of a number of years.

The inside of my head feels scorched, the way our eyes get from staring at the sun. It's always like this: a light too bright to be tolerated has shone into every cell of my brain and I can't see, have spots of un-thought floating across my mind. Dragging the words I want to say, one at a time, out of the storage bins of words is exhausting, as if each one weighs a ton.

Then there are the muscles. In those few seconds of wildness, they have contracted hard enough to crack stone. They have clenched beyond anything I could do with my waking will. Every strand hurts. My sacrum is jammed, my right hip excruciating, my left knee and ankle pulled awry. My arms, my back, my thighs, my face— it's as if each separate part of me climbed its own mountain range and is aching from the labor of it. It's as if I was beaten up from the inside. I'm all bruise.

The storm no longer strikes without warning, or rather, I've become a storm reader. Instead of green skies and tornado sirens, I begin to have trouble retrieving words. Someone speaks, and there's a long delay before I understand what was said and can begin to reach for an answer. It means parts of my brain are already flickering on the edge of the hyper-coordinated dance that will sweep in and take over from lovely randomness.

I recognized the storm warnings on Wednesday, but it had been four years since I had a knock-down, drag-out seizure and I was cocky. I even had a visitation. A beautiful blue jay perched on a branch outside my window, and I told my helper, "that's my mother." The bird began to peck at a branch and I said, "she's telling me to eat," but I didn't do it. I thought lying down and sipping passionflower tonic would be enough. So after a while I got up and went to the dining room. The last thing I remember is standing facing the fridge. The next thing I remember is my niece saying, "she died."

I learned to recognize my danger zones from a woman named Donna Andrews who not only woke herself from a vegetative state, but learned how to stop her ten seizures a day, some forty years ago, and with neurologist Joel Reiter, developed a protocol for teaching others. She taught me to listen to my body, to recognize the risk factors unique to my being, to know where the limits of safety lie, for me. In the last six years I've stopped many seizures, identifying what stressors were dragging me toward that edge and reducing them, one by one, until my brain no longer needed to throw an emergency switch.

But in the last few months, stressors have piled up one on top of another and my ability to know how I'm doing has been numbed. Donna always told me I could go out on one limb or two but not three. I was out on about five limbs last Wednesday, without knowing it.

I cultivate awareness of the subtle states of my bodymind in many ways. I control my immediate environment as much as I can, so that I notice changes. I make my room a sanctuary, where subtle shifts will show up against a soothing background. I retreat to my introvert's cave at the first hint of over-stimulation. Sleep, food, exertion, temperature, emotion, sensory input, a build-up of stories. These are the compass points, the factors whose levels I must be aware of. If I'm not sleeping well, I have to eat extra carefully. If I'm upset, I need to rest and stretch. If

I am collecting stories, I have to write them, give them away before they pile up in my head and trigger an avalanche.

But half my belongings are 3,500 miles away and I can't find that red velour sweater, or the golden mask of the Epileptic Ancestor that I've been working on. I packed up a 35 year life and drove across the continent to my father in the hospital, in and out and in again, half a dozen times, had barely unpacked before I was flying home to Puerto Rico for the first time in six years, learned something shocking while I was there that interrupted my sleep for weeks, and also felt more drawn to live there than ever before (excitement is as dangerous as being upset), came back to more medical emergencies and unpacking, all the while moving into my mother's room, moving her belongings out, then drove to Albany, cocky still, I suppose, from my cross country trek, gave a talk and got food poisoning and had to be fetched because I was too sick to drive. For the last few weeks my father was extremely anxious, his worries confused and repetitive, and I spent my waking hours talking him down from ledges, my adrenaline sky high around the clock. There wasn't enough help and I was on all the time. My fine tuned sensors got overwhelmed and after four years and a carefully built up buffer zone, I thought I was safe. But I spent it all down in three hectic months.

This is where the model mugging metaphor is more accurate than it seems. My body was in fact acting in my best defense, protecting me from unbearable levels of stress by blowing a circuit, like those little red buttons in bathrooms. My beautiful, sensitive brain threw itself on the assailants, did those model mugging moves without my conscious participation, and left me to read the hospital reports.

Patients

Why do they call us "the patient"

We are not patient. We endure.

The anxious tedium of public hospital

waiting rooms, because waiting

is the punishment of the poor;

interminable buses to inconvenient places

where we count up our cash, calculating

whether we can take a cab home

instead of riding our exhaustion;

the angry contempt of specialists, taught to believe

any pain they cannot explain is insubordinate,

deliberate, offensive.

We are not patient. We are denied.

Not medically necessary, they say, not proven.

Feel free to appeal. We are experts at appealing,

so we begin again, gathering documents, faxing releases,

collecting letters and signatures,

giving our numbers, all our numbers,

to dozens of indifferent, underpaid clerks,

stacking up evidence for the hearing,

where we will declare

as civilly as we can to the affronted panels

that it is necessary that we breathe,

sleep, digest, be eased of pain, have medicines

and therapies and machines,

and that we not be required to beg.

While I am waiting, I am using my pen,

steadily altering words.

Where the card says "medically indigent"

I cross it out and write *indignant.*

Where my records say "chemically sensitive"

I write *chemically assaulted, chemically wounded,*

chemically outraged. On the form listing risk factors

for cancer, I write in my candidates: agribusiness,

air fresheners, dry cleaning, river water, farm life,

bathing, drinking, eating, vinyl, cosmetics, plastic, greed.

I am making an intricate graffiti poem

out of mountains of unnecessary paperwork.

Where the doctor has written "disheveled"

I write *untamed.*

Where it says "refused treatment", I write

refused to be lied to.

Where it says safe, side effects minimal

I say *prove it. What do you mean minimal?*

What do you mean side? I write

unmarketed effects unmentionable.

Where it asks, authorization? I write *inherent,*

authorized from birth.

Are you the patient? she asks, ready to transfer my call.

I say *only with my own sweet, brave body.*

I say, *Not today, no. I have no patience left.*

I am the person who is healing, I say,

in spite of everything.

I will have to put you on hold she says. *Yes,*

hold me I say. *That would be good.*

Some Thoughts on Environmental Illness

This article was originally written for the Re-evaluation Counseling Communities (RC) which I have been part of since 1984. RC is an international network of peer counselors committed to reclaiming our flexible intelligence and full humanity from the effects of having been hurt, and to ending all forms of humans harming each other and the environment. "Distress" refers to patterns of thoughts, feelings and behaviors that are the result of being hurt, a kind of psychological scar tissue, that, like physical scars, are rigid and constrict free movement. Distress patterns do not represent our best thinking about the actual present moment, but can be quite convincing. All forms of oppression, including internalized oppression, are distress patterns. "Discharge" refers to the natural physical processes that release stress and dissolve the effects of hurt so that we remain flexible in spite of painful experiences. Discharge includes crying, shaking, raging, yawning, sweating and rapid, non-repetitive taking. "Directions" are phrases, thoughts, or physical actions used in counseling sessions to bring about discharge. You can learn more about RC at www.rc.org

Misconceptions About EI

There are many widespread misconceptions about environmental illness, also known as multiple chemical sensitivity, the most widespread of which is that it's imaginary—or, in RC terms, that it's purely the expression of distress recordings and has no physical basis. This is similar to the way many people thought about Chronic Fatigue Immune Dysfunction Syndrome until recently, when more sophisticated research began showing clear evidence of what patients had been reporting for decades. (For instance, people with CFIDS have been saying for years that exercise makes us feel worse. Recent research shows that the bodies of people with CFIDS really do react differently to exercise. A molecule that marks levels of pain and tiredness rises four times as much in people with CFIDS, and lasts for several days, instead of a few hours.)

Environmental Illness is understood by the people who study it to be a complex response by many different systems in the body to the immense increase in the number and amounts of poison in our environment during the last 75 years. How each sick person responds depends on which systems in their bodies are weakest, what chemicals they have been exposed to, what resources they have, and what other hardships and distresses they face in their lives.

There's a belief that the people who get EI are mostly white, class privileged and have irrational beliefs about reality, of which their illness is one. In fact, people of color worldwide suffer from much higher levels of exposure to toxins, and have significantly less access to health care. In the US, medical practitioners who diagnose and work with EI tend to be holistic doctors who don't accept insurance and are out of the reach of the majority of people of color. Environmental illnesses affect many people in poor neighborhoods, but are described differently (as asthma, migraines, allergies, etc.) or never diagnosed at all.

There is a belief that because discharge or other emotional work sometimes improves EI symptoms, this proves that the symptoms were not physical, and that people who don't recover just haven't done enough work. Discharge helps all situations. In the case of physical illness, that can include improving symptoms or just giving us more ability to think well about ourselves. Discharge can make a broken bone hurt less and heal faster. That doesn't mean the bone wasn't broken. Discharge adds resilience to our systems, and sometimes that allows the body to better fight off illness. That doesn't mean the illness was not physical or real, only that for that individual, discharge was one of the things that allowed the body's healing abilities to work better, and the improvement was enough to change their symptoms. Another person might do just as much emotional work, and the effect of that might not change their symptoms, just how they think about their experience, or what medical choices they make.

Physical or Emotional is Political

Whether a set of symptoms is seen by the oppressive society as physical or psychological depends on many non-medical factors. Science has increasingly shown that, in fact, all illnesses and distresses have both physical and psychological aspects, and in many cases, they're hard to tell apart. Emotional states are also chemical states, thought can change brain structure and function, hormone levels change our emotions, etc. Whenever anyone is adamant that a malfunction of our complex body-mind is 100% physical or 100% psychological it's because oppression is involved. Either the oppression itself needs us to understand the problem in a certain way in order to continue, or people are resisting oppression in rigid and reactive ways.

The current U.S. medical system often sees depression as 100% a chemical imbalance and treats it with drugs, while it often sees environmental illness as psychological and recommends psychotherapy. If there was widespread recognition that many people are depressed because oppression makes us miserable, and that large numbers of people are getting sick because of the reckless use of toxic chemicals for profit, more of us might become inspired to organize, and resist the policies that make us sick and sad.

And because of the tremendous harm done by psychiatric drugs, people who resist their use sometimes rigidly insist that our physical bodies—hormones, neurotransmitters, nutrients, brain tissue—are never the causes of our mental states. This doesn't make any sense, when we know that, for example, injecting someone with adrenaline will make them agitated, and touching certain areas of the brain with a probe can make someone feel happy, sad, or angry.

For a short time, many years ago, I became extremely depressed once a month for a single day. During that one day I felt suicidal. It turned out that this was always on the same day of my menstrual cycle, a day when my progesterone levels should have gone up and didn't. The content of my depression came from my own history and my specific distress patterns, but it was set off by low progesterone combined with some other medical conditions that made me especially sensitive to changes in hormone levels. I started using progesterone cream, and the mid-cycle depression vanished. I needed to discharge the early hurts that were the content of the depression, and I also needed progesterone to stop those distresses from expressing themselves strongly on the same day of my cycle every month.

On the other hand, because people with some of the newer chronic illnesses have been treated very badly, with the excuse that our symptoms are believed to be purely psychological, some people in the EI community insist there are no psychological reasons for our illness at all. I don't know if this is true, but it seems to me that an unusually high number of people with EI have had traumatic experiences like sexual abuse early in their lives. This is also true of many people who aren't sick with EI, but for this example, let's agree that a higher than usual number of people with EI were abused as children, and that one result is a distress pattern of feeling that the world is dangerous and that we can't protect ourselves.

That doesn't in any way change the reality that toxic exposures can overpower our immune systems and make us sick, and it doesn't "prove" that EI is a purely emotional response to trauma. There are many possible ways to understand how emotional trauma is connected to immune systems not working well. What I think is that early extreme hurts, and the distress patterns of fear and vigilance they can leave behind, interfere with our immune systems so that they become over-reactive and don't do as good a job of defending us against the many dangerous toxins we get exposed to; that toxins and distresses combined can overwhelm our bodies' defenses, and that each one makes us more vulnerable to the other. What it does not mean is that people whose immune systems are affected by trauma have physical symptoms because they haven't tried hard enough.

My Personal Story: What I Was Exposed To and How It Affected Me

I was born on a farm in Puerto Rico, in 1954, during a period when large amounts of toxic chemicals were being promoted as a modern and better way to live. Many of these chemicals had been developed as weapons and the companies that made them were looking for ways to sell them after WWII ended. Many of the pesticides used on our farm started out as nerve gases used in war. US companies sold those chemicals to Puerto Rican farmers, the government promoted them, and some of them ended up being made in my country without good enough protection for workers or the environment.

I was also sexually abused in extreme ways during the time I was in elementary school, by a group of men connected to my school, and my parents were targeted for being communists. I experienced a lot of fear growing up. Starting around the age of nine I began having pains in my legs and getting out of breath going up hills. When we moved to Chicago, when I was thirteen, I started having throat and respiratory infections, and was so tired I had a hard time walking even a few blocks. During my adult life, I have had better and worse times, but overall, I have gotten sicker. When I became pregnant with my daughter, her father and I moved into a home that had new carpets, paint, adhesives, and other chemicals, and I became very sick. I started reacting strongly to household chemicals, perfumes and natural gas. I also started having pain in my liver, even though the usual tests didn't show any problems. Eventually I became so weak and tired and had so much pain that I was unable to continue working.

For many years I felt very bad about myself for being sick. No one could explain why I was so tired, and why I got sick when I was around scented products. I was often mistreated for being ill. People told me I was misbehaving, demanding attention by having symptoms that were just dramatic performances of my distress patterns. I was told I was lazy, lying, just wanted to avoid working, was making a fuss about nothing. Many people thought that if laundry detergent perfumes didn't make everyone equally sick, they couldn't really be making me sick. Constantly being told that what I experienced wasn't real, and worse, was a sign of bad behavior, made me defensive, so that it was hard to calmly ask for what I needed.

Three years ago I saw a new doctor who knew how to interpret a recently developed genetic test I'd had done some time before. It turns out that nine of my liver enzymes, responsible for breaking down and removing toxins from my body, don't do what they're supposed to because of genetic differences from normal enzymes. She told me that one or two such defects could cause all the symptoms I have, and that with nine of them, it's no surprise that I have epilepsy, migraines, pain and inflammation in my muscles and joints, strange reactions to many drugs, and get very sick from laundry detergent fragrance, cigarette smoke, diesel fumes, and fresh paint. Because my body can't get rid of toxins the way it needs to, they pile up in my body and make me extremely sensitive to new ones.

I found out that one of the pesticides I was exposed to as a child is used to create epilepsy in lab rats. The process, called kindling, is one of the current explanations for EI. Given enough stress to the brain, for instance extreme hunger, thirst, fatigue, altitude or emotional shock, anyone can have a seizure. Small, repeated doses of toxic chemicals change the brain so that it takes much less to set off seizures. This is what they do to the lab rats, so they can test anti-seizure medications on them. I had repeated small doses of pesticides that kill insects by damaging their nervous systems. Because my liver doesn't get rid of such poisons very well, I was more likely to be kindled by pesticides than most people. Once people are kindled, smaller changes have bigger effects.

Some scientists believe that this is what causes people to get EI. They get exposed to small doses of many poisonous chemicals, and if they are more vulnerable, for any reason, they start reacting to small amounts of poison as if they were large amounts. I have no doubt that emotional trauma is one reason why people, and rats, are vulnerable to kindling.

Infectious Disease is Our Model for Illness

Our medical system developed through the fight against infectious diseases. With infections, one microbe causes more or less the same symptoms in all people, and all people with that disease get it from the same cause. But the newer chronic illnesses that have appeared or become much more common in the recent period (EI, CFIDS, Fibromyalgia) often have many causes, and can show up differently in different people, which makes it very hard for medical science to figure out what to do about them. We're exposed to tens of thousands of newly created toxic molecules that our bodies have no experience with. There are thousands of chemicals that affect our nervous systems, but how our nervous systems respond to poisons varies depending on genetics, distresses, environment and what else is happening.

It's easy for some people to get dizzy and have blurred vision, nausea and swollen glands from being in the garden section of a hardware store, while someone else has the exact same symptoms from laundry products, and a third person responds to the same exposure with muscle weakness, twitching limbs, tingling and numbness in their fingers, and mental confusion. In order to understand these illnesses, we have to pay attention to all the ways our bodies and minds and emotions interact and respond to threats. But our medical system isn't set up to do this. People who treat the nervous system are in a different part of the hospital from people who treat the immune system or work with hormones. And most doctors don't pay attention to how distress affects our bodies. If they notice that this is the case, they send us to a "mental health" specialist.

How Chronic Illness is Different from Disability

People with chronic illness experience some of the same oppression as people with physical disabilities, and the two groups have sometimes been allies in fighting that oppression (defending access to health care and social services, insisting on access to education and services, fighting for respect of our bodies as they are.) But our experiences are different in important ways. Most people with physical disabilities know exactly what their disability is. Like infectious diseases, most disabilities have a single known cause. Many people with disabilities are healthy. They have different physical limits than currently able bodied people, but they are not sick.

Some disabled people have conditions that get worse over time, and of course they can feel better and worse like everyone else, but in most cases, their condition doesn't change dramatically from day to day. People with the chronic illnesses that affect many systems, like EI, don't usually know exactly what is causing us to be sick. The same symptoms can have different causes, and how sick we are can vary a lot. Healthy people find this confusing. They think that "real" sickness is consistent. If the symptoms change from day to day, they can't be real. People often argue with us, telling us that they used the same scented soap last month and we didn't get headaches then, so it can't be the soap that is making our heads hurt today. That's not how our bodies work. Last month we got enough sleep, our neighbor who smokes was away on vacation, and it was warm, so we didn't have to turn on the furnace. This month the smoker is back, the furnace is leaking small amounts of fumes into our bedrooms and we're not sleeping very well, so the small extra challenge of the perfumed soap is enough to cause a headache. Our symptoms aren't consistent, but our bodies make sense.

I have a close friend who has a form of Muscular Dystrophy called Infantile Progressive Spinal Muscular Atrophy. She is in a wheelchair and her muscles are too weak for her to lift her arms by herself or pick up objects. Her disability is obvious to anyone who sees her, and her challenge is to get people to understand that she is powerful and competent. On bad days, I am unable to get out of my bed, it takes all my energy to get to the bathroom, all my muscles and joints hurt, and a small amount of fragrance makes my whole body react strongly. But no-one can tell by looking at me. My challenge is to get people to understand that I have a real struggle. My friend's oppression pushes her to hide her struggles and always act strong and speak powerfully in order to be treated as human. Mine pushes me both ways—I have to show my struggles and insist that my condition is serious in order to get help, but I also get mistreated for needing that help. Most healthy people assume I am exaggerating when I tell my story, when in fact I am usually showing them only a small part of what I struggle with.

Because we're more used to thinking about infectious diseases as a model of sickness, and wheelchair users as a model of disability, and because people with complicated chronic illnesses don't fit either model, it's hard, even for those who love us to understand our experience. Most often, this takes the form of not believing us. As a society, our thinking about bodies, emotions and minds has been artificially split apart, and people are blamed for pain that is thought to be emotional, while pain that is thought to be physical is usually not seen as our fault. (Some people do get blamed for physical pain, for instance people with AIDS are sometimes targeted in this way.) Because symptoms that are not understood are usually assumed to be caused by distress or to be "psychiatric," people like me get targeted with mental health oppression for describing physical suffering that doesn't fit neatly into our usual models of sickness.

Why We Continue To Use Toxic Products

In the US, cosmetics and many household products aren't regulated. The corporations that make them don't have to tell us what's in them and there's no law preventing manufacturers from knowingly including toxic ingredients. An activist scientist recently did an analysis of the ingredients in a popular detergent with a strongly scented fabric softener as part of its formula. It turned out to have over 500 ingredients, including 28 known to cause cancer and many others proven to damage the nervous system or interfere with hormone balance, which can cause serious problems for growing children. When my body reacts to fabric softener by giving me nausea, headaches, twitching muscles, confusion, blurred vision, flu symptoms, and aching joints, this is just a sped up and amplified version of what those chemicals do to everyone. There are similarly dangerous chemicals in many shampoos, deodorants, colognes, cosmetics used on our eyes and lips, and other popular products.

These products are made by workers who get exposed to high concentrations of harmful chemicals every day. These same chemicals contaminate our water, soil and air while they are being made, while they're being used, and when they wash down the drain into our rivers and lakes, or end up in landfill in discarded containers.

When this information is made available to people, we might expect them to appreciate the warning and quickly change the products they use, in order to protect their health. Instead, they often become angry with those who tell them, usually people who suffer from EI, and that anger often takes the form of insisting that we're making it up and imposing our irrational beliefs on them. The industries that make and sell these products tap into a powerful set of distresses about how our homes and bodies smell. The oppression of people of the global majority, Jews, and poor people, among others, include specific misinformation that says we're dirty and smell bad. Women are assaulted with constant messages that our bodies are wrong and must be fixed in order for us to be valued at all, and that includes being told to spray strong chemicals on our vaginas and armpits to change how they smell, and to constantly perfume our hair and skin, our clothing, our dishes, and our floors with chemicals that will make them smell "fresh."

Because of the many ways we've all been made to feel bad about ourselves, we have distressed attachments to perfumes and "favorite" brands of products that are extremely toxic to all people, bad for the environment and cause suffering and isolation for those of us whose bodies react faster to poison.

Why We Should Stop

There is no rational reason for anyone to ever use these products again, and ending their use moves us forward on many liberation goals at once. Within RC we have the tools and understanding to allow us to discharge our feelings that these products provide us with something important, that giving them up is a hardship, and that by asking you to stop using them, people with EI are behaving inappropriately, or making unreasonable demands.

The impact on those of us who are sick is very big. My body's reactivity to widely used toxins means every time I get on an airplane I risk being seated next to someone drenched in perfume. If that happens, I can lose control of my limbs, be unable to speak, get blurred vision and dizziness, nausea and a headache, have trouble breathing, and have seizures, which can cause serious injuries and even be life threatening. I can't stay in hotels or most private homes. I'm unable to attend most RC workshops because the sites we use are not chemically accessible, and most members of our communities have not discharged enough on these issues to decide to be chemically safe. Entering a room full of people who use conventional laundry products, with a carpet that's been cleaned with chemical rug cleaner, is dangerous for me.

I'm unable to have face to face sessions except with the very few people who have decided to stop using any scented products at all, and have gone through the process of removing leftover chemicals from their clothing. (Laundry perfume is deliberately engineered to stick to fabric for a long time, and has to be removed by repeatedly washing clothing in baking soda, borax, and/or vinegar.) **What isolates me is not my illness, but the widespread distress that prevents people from choosing non-toxic products, for their own sake, for the world, and in order to be close to people like me.**

I know that being physically and sexually abused as a young person made me vulnerable to my immune and nervous systems becoming overwhelmed. I know that my genetic liver condition, and my exposure to pesticides based on nerve gas, also set me up to be ill. I continue to discharge about the early abuse, the pesticide exposure, my liver condition, and what it feels like to have people who I know care about me be unwilling to change their brand of detergent or shampoo for my sake. I continue to discharge the feelings of defensiveness, humiliation, shame and fear that many people with EI experience.

I'm able, now, to talk about this as a liberation issue that affects us all, and to invite the RC communities to take this on, not as a favor to me, but as an act of resistance to our manipulation, to the destruction of our environment and to capitalism's assault on our bodies, and an act of solidarity with those of us who, for many different reasons, are hit faster and harder by the poisons that eventually affect us all.

Some Possible Directions for Discharge

What would you have to face if you decided environmental illness is real, and affects everyone?

What would you have to face if you decided to stop using all scented products? Try the decision. What feelings come up?

Thinking about environmental illness leads to thinking about how oppression is poisoning our environment. What comes up for you when you consider the environmental toxicity created by oppression?

When did you first hear about people becoming sick from environmental toxins? How did you feel? What did you assume to be true about it? Do you know anyone with environmental illness? How do you feel about their condition?

Many people with environmental illness also have a lot of food allergies. Most of us were hurt as young people by being forced to eat food we didn't like, and may have internalized oppressor patterns like "Eat what's on your plate," and "Don't be so picky." What was your early relationship to food choices?

What's your experience with chronic illness? Who was the first chronically sick person you met and how did you feel about them?

Have you ever been told you were faking a physical condition, were a hypochondriac, or were making too much of a fuss about a physical condition? What was that like?

Have you ever ignored a physical condition because of fear of how you would be treated if you acknowledged it?

Stricken

First poem written after my 2007 stroke, which took all day to type

what a dish

half woman

half noodle.

most people prefer that she top herself

with something creamy

and cheerfully mild

worried she might be

frightfully bitter

or just frightening.

secretly

she is chewing arugula

and dandelion greens

into a stinging pesto

of bad attitude.

staring at a can she wonders

can she train her teeth

to chomp around the edges?

life is no zip top.

dexterity comes from dexter

to be adroit in a right handed world.

who knew it took such intricate cooperation

to floss your teeth?

she imagines the millions who knew

wielding one handed toothpicks

stringing thread between their toes

refusing to surrender their mouths.

she tries to write

but her hand pours itself

all over the keyboard

spills between the space bar

and the letter N.

she wakes up tied to her muscles

feeling like lead,

hating how the sun

calls to her through the curtains.

nothing has prepared her

to do nothing

but be.

she feels disobedient

or shallow

for not feeling enlightened.

the shallowest river she's ever seen

was the Gale river, only a hand span of ice green water

gurgling between hard, delicate

winter glass above, and a bed of stones.

through that narrow translucent space

mountain water, achingly cold,

made silent eddies—

graceful, frozen curls of white,

across the river's face.

she imagines herself

a twig twisting through gaps between rocks,

a one legged newt buried in bottom mud.

Already it's time for lunch,

bowl held tight to the apron covered chest

in the crook of the weak arm, held up with pillows,

dipping a spoon with the strong left hand

that doesn't know how.

in the afternoons she listens to spring birds in the oaks

lies very still on her bed

moves fingers, legs, toes in her mind

feeling nerves tingle

with the force of her will for them

at night she dreams

she is picking up tiny blue beads

dropping them one by one

into a black bowl

impulses of light

in a curve of silence.

Stroke: A Dance Performance

This poem was the sound track to a dance piece I performed for the Sins Invalid 2011 Showcase, in which I told the story of my stroke rehab, and the complete absence of any attention to sexuality as a part of stroke recovery.

stroke

stroke

stroke

when it happened,

the right side of my body disappeared from the map

left only tangled lines. Everything dragged down towards earth

except for my pinkie that curled up and out like a twig.

when it happened, my foot was pierced with fire,

but cold and swollen

as waterlogged wood.

my skin couldn't bear the weight of my sheets.

touch made me scream and weep.

when it happened, my hand was scalded, wracked with spasms,

a dense slab of pain. Five fingers set adrift from my brain

couldn't cup, grip, press, pinch.

therapy began with holding my right foot in my left hand

and squeezing

so it would know where it was. so the crazy screaming nerves

would calm down and remember to be *foot*.

therapy was holding my runaway fingers together

reuniting the pinkie with the ring finger,

teaching them to be *hand*.

therapy was stepping on needles, on burning asphalt,

on glaciers. ten steps. fifteen. try again.

start rubbing the skin with silk, they said,

with wool

with terry cloth

put sandpaper on the toilet seat.

apply texture to the hypersensitive and the dulled.

the arm, the hand, the leg, the foot, the face.

no one asked, no one ever asked

about inner skin

about silk and touch and stiff

uno dos tres cuatro cinco

all summer at the gym in Havana

all day every day step and step and step

up down open close

my hand clenching, spreading, uncurling

my foot stepping, bending, arching

walking

strongly

on the earth

but no one asked, no one ever asked

do you feel this?

the injured brain forgets the places it's lost connection with,

blank spaces in the atlas, unexplored oceans

find your missing continents, they said

grasp with your hand, put weight on your foot, touch your face,

use it or lose it.

but no one asked

do you feel this?

or this?

no one said,

pleasure is a lost continent

touch yourself with silk

how is your clitoris today?

use it or lose it.

stroke, stroke, stroke

no one helps me.

I explore the dry places and the wetlands.

struggle to clench and release muscles that forgot how.

rub dry sticks trying to raise a spark.

open, close, open, close

tracing the tips of nerves that have been sleeping

hoping they will wake up and remember to be delicious

the hand that dives in is still thick as a novacained cheek.

it cramps on the vibrator.

how do I tell which is numb,

the slick, ridged wall or the finger.

clench and release, clench and release

breath takes me down

breath is a bridge across numbness

closing gaps in the circuits

streaming past burnt neurons

chi dancing naked in the dead places

becomes my instructor

exercise imagination she murmurs,

remember

wet tongue, long finger, velvet cock

breathe them into bound muscle

conjure sensation out of thin air.

the imprint of memory

begins restoring the coastline of pleasure

mirages shimmer in the air, forgotten peaks

floating above flesh

breathe them in

breathe them out

become what I have lost

until nothing is missing

stroke

stroke

stroke

stroke

stroke

Coming Out Sick

Living with my father, for the first time I am managing my health in full view of a family member. Until she moved out at eighteen, my daughter lived with my chronic illness and the series of catastrophic crises it routinely generates. She had to navigate the choppy seas of a childhood full of emergencies and the vast doldrums of my exhaustion, inevitably more of a caretaker than she should have had to be.

In that world of impending shipwrecks, avoiding the tips of icebergs was enough to handle. The deep, cold, roots of my condition, the massive flanks and fissures, were places I went alone, in the dark, filling notebooks in sleepless nights of poring over self-help books and websites and list-serves organized by shared and overlapping diagnoses, drafting new protocols, (liver cleansing, chelation, alkalinity, rotation diets, EMF shielding) looking for explanations, or at least relief, consulting one narrowly focused healer after another, trying out the pills, potions and practices that resonated, tracking changes (seizures, menstrual cycles, sleep and appetite and pain, mood swings, dreams, the clarity of my mind,) traveling by sonar.

The people by my bedside saw the cups of bitter tea and bowls of pills, but not the insomniac research behind them.

I am living with my father for the first time since I was sixteen. Not since the full-impact years of single motherhood have I had this much responsibility for another person's well-being, and I'm drowning, unable to balance his needs and my own, both of us in shock at our changed worlds since my mother died and I uprooted myself to come here. I am struggling to exercise self care, which is hard enough without this balancing act, hard enough when no one's watching up close, seeing each choice I make.

For decades I have studied my body and its responses, learned what helps and what doesn't. I have encyclopedic knowledge of the effects of nutrients, herbs, externally applied substances and internal energy practices, am adept at adding micrograms of this and that to the scales, balancing pain relief with a need for alertness, the adrenal boost and the sleeping potion. Tonight I introduce him to the plants we both take as bedtime tinctures, show him pictures of long-standing allies, the companions I've turned to in pain-wracked nights and sleepless pre-dawns. The purple bells of skullcap, periwinkle stars of vervain, maroon and yellow blossom of wild stream orchid.

I tell him that last night I was drenched in sweat. Do I know why he asks. I explain that I live at the hub of multiple diagnoses, where symptoms criss-cross and can be claimed by any of a handful of causes. Night sweats can be Bartonella or Babesia, two of the co-infections of Lyme, or CFIDS, that uncharted sea of devastating neuro-immune dysfunction that some people still insist is hysteria. Adrenal stress alone can drench the sheets.

We've just watched an episode of The West Wing in which President Bartlett has an MS attack. The First Lady wipes down his damp brow, says gently that he's sweated through his clothes, and the Surgeon General explains to the gathered staff that tiring himself could lead to spasms of his legs. Suddenly my eyes fill with tears. The severity of my illness has been dawning on me in a new way, again. I, too, sweat through my clothes, wake up in damp sheets, and for the last two years, the muscles of my calves and feet have gone into frequent, excruciating spasm. I don't know much about MS, what the relationship is between demyelination and sweat, but my own MRIs show a multitude of "punctate areas of high signal intensity" in the white matter of my brain. Maybe it's the scars in the white matter that are making me sweat.

The constellations of lesions in my brain are interpreted differently by each specialist who looks at them. Like astronomers from different cultures, they impose their own meanings, seeing different pictures in the patterns of light and dark, the Dipper or the Great Bear, Lyra or Weaving Girl, a rabbit or an old man in the stains of shadow on the moon. Those splotches revealed by magnetic resonance have been explained to me as degenerative vascular disease, multiple sclerosis, the scars of dozens of seizures, the tracks of Lyme or Bartonella or both, the wreckage left by hundreds of complicated migraine episodes constricting blood flow, or whatever it is that allows CFIDS to damage the brain. Like the classic fable of the blind men and the elephant, no one can offer me a complete picture.

But in the highly politicized, profit driven worlds of the medical industry and the labyrinths of publicly funded social services, which of the overlapping diagnoses I pursue, and in what order, and in whose view, may ultimately be a strategic, rather than a medical decision. The symptoms may be the same, but it's easier to get resources under some identities than others. After thirty years of advocacy and research, it may be better, at least officially, to have CFIDS than chronic Lyme, a diagnosis that has lost physicians their licenses in some states, and is at the center of a raging war for profit, power and prestige.

So, late into my insomniac night, I revisit CFIDS after a few years of doing my suffering under other names. What strikes me is the accumulation, in recent years, of solid evidence not only that CFIDS is a physical, measurable illness, but also documenting its severity. After decades of ridicule and dismissal, it's been less exhausting to downplay the intensity of how sick I feel, then to deal with the emotional battering of people's skepticism, the assumption that this is attention seeking melodrama, the endless unsolicited recommendations of everything from chamomile tea to affirmations. But I think the worst of it is my inability to tell the truth of what I experience without feeling like every word must be a gross exaggeration, when in fact it's usually a serious understatement.

In a 2010 speech, leading CFIDS researcher Dr. Anthony Komaroff cites a major study on the severity of CFIDS, using a research survey called the SF-36, considered one of the best tools for measuring how sick people are. When compared to subjects with heart failure and depression, CFIDS patients had a physical status similar to heart failure patients, the highest levels of pain and lowest levels of vitality and social functioning of all three groups, and substantially better mental health than the depressed patients. Another study looked for physiological evidence of the wiped out feeling known as "post-exertional malaise," comparing levels of molecules that detect pain and fatigue in CFIDS patients and healthy controls. For the healthy subjects, the levels peak eight hours after exercising, at two and half times the pre-exercise level. For those with CFIDS, the levels continue to climb until they are nine times higher than normal, and they stay that way up to 48 hours after exercising.

These are only two among many studies cited, and reading them is like suddenly discovering that I've been granted citizenship, and can come out of hiding. I feel vindicated, like a crime victim whose testimony is finally believed. And then, browsing through the introduction to Peggy Munson's ground breaking anthology Stricken, I find this:

> "Dr. Mark Loveless, an infectious disease specialist, proclaimed that a CFIDS patient 'feels every day significantly the same as an AIDS patient feels two months before death.'"

I have a dear friend who is facing a second bout of ovarian cancer, an exquisite being whose honesty and vulnerability, courage and humor, affect me like the most potent of my medicinal tinctures, an essence of integrity. When she writes, I write back, even when I'm very ill. This week I wrote to her about the words "terminal" and "interminable" side by side, about life-threatening and life-draining as categories of illness. When my mother was in her last several years of living with multiple myeloma, she would call me for advice on how to live with such exhaustion, how to cope with such limited energy, such restricted capacity, and I would tell her how I do it. I held her hand while she passed through the territory I live in, and on out of life. Now I live in the room she died in, and I'm still exhausted.

Although people with CFIDS, Environmental Illness and similar conditions have a high rate of suicide, and epileptics are six times more likely to be seriously depressed than healthy people, I am fully committed to being alive. But there's an intensity of suffering for millions of us, that most people have no idea of, and the crazy-making result of its invisibility is that at the same time that I'm struggling to tender my body and soul the very best loving care I can, silently affirming my capacity to heal, all the while that I'm trying to live as fully and joyously as I can within these states of exhausted pain— in order to protect myself from complete collapse, in order to get access to even minimal support and ridiculously inadequate care, I have write on form after form, chant loudly and continuously to agencies and authorities, acquaintances, family and friends: I'm sick, I'm sick, I'm sick.

I have another dear friend whose body instantly declares her disability to the world, who must fight to be seen as competent, while I fight to be seen as needing help. Within the ever-shifting dynamics of capacity and incapacity, illness and health, vulnerability and strength, each of us holds truths that are partly submerged. I know my survival depends on communicating both my competence and incompetence, my resilience and know-how, and my stark limitations; that I have to hold my own and surrender, accept limits and push against them.

So this is what I'm thinking about these days, days that fall away from the clock, when I sleep from dawn to noon, or, like today, from midnight to 5 am. How to be publicly sick and empowered. How to bring my whole self into view and still be safe, supported. How to be sick and undiagnosed and unashamed; or over-diagnosed, in a storm of contradictory instructions and stories, and stay calm, accepting uncertainty. How to shed the million ways I am named by others and just be. How to wear my own face.

CUBA

A Day in the Life

Monday, May 4, 2009 10:45 am.
Social Security Office, Berkeley, CA

It takes an hour and half, even with the help of a very friendly social worker, to fill out all the paperwork on my application for disability benefits and Medicare. I turned fifty-five in February and the premiums on my already costly insurance shot up to $1200 a month. Even with all my papers in order, and clear evidence that I have not been able to work for three years, it will take another year before the government starts paying for a portion of my medical expenses, which overshadow every other item in my budget.

I tell the social worker that I will be out of the country for two months.

"Where are you going?"

"Cuba. For medical treatment."

Unlike many of the people I've told, he doesn't ask why. Instead he says, "How fantastic!" He hears they have great medical care. I wish now that I'd asked him how he knew—from seeing Sicko? From listening to KPFA? Because our congresswoman, Barbara Lee, is one of the sponsors of a bill to lift the travel ban? Just living in Berkeley isn't enough. Over and over people have looked at me blankly. "Cuba? Why?" Today someone asked me, "What do they have that we don't have here?"

For a year I have been reading and rereading the website of CIREN, the International Center for Neurological Restoration. On bad days, on days when I'm driven mad by the fragmented nature of my health care, with a specialist for each separate molecule of me, when I am aghast at the unselfconscious arrogance and contempt with which most medical doctors regard the healing practices of other traditions and cultures, when I start tallying up the real costs, spiritual and emotional as well as physical and economic, of being a patient in this particularly ferocious manifestation of late stage capitalism, when I'm shaken with rage at the sheer cruelty of what is denied to sick people in this country, I go to the CIREN website.

For a very long time now, I have had severe Chronic Fatigue Immune Dysfunction Syndrome, that mysterious collection of devastating symptoms that the dominant medical practices of our country have no idea what to do with. Three years ago I collapsed while on a speaking tour and have been unable to work ever since. A month later I fell during an epileptic seizure and had a moderate brain injury, from which it took a year to recover. Two years ago I had a stroke, and can no longer walk more than thirty or forty feet, so I use a power wheelchair to get around. After the allotted number of once a week, forty-five minute physical therapy sessions authorized by my health plan had been used up, there was nothing else on offer. To get rehab you have to be in that window of need where you continue to show easily measured improvement, and have easily measured remaining deficits, of the type that there are easily mobilized plans to deal with. If you reach a plateau, you get pushed off.

One day last fall I realized I wasn't willing to settle for what I had. One reason was the story of my friend Teresa Walsh. Following a spinal cord injury from a fall, she, too, went as far as the insurance would take her, and was told that being in a wheelchair for the rest of her life was as healed as she would get. Her story about her decision to go Cuba for care was told in her own one-woman show. When both the disbelief about my stroke, and the joy of wheelchair mobility started to wear off, it was her story I thought of. I just woke up one day with a wish that had become a decision: I'm going to Cuba.

My father has been training Cuban ecologists for nearly forty-five years. Until two years ago, he went every February for several weeks, and he has many friends and colleagues there. He was the one who told me about CIREN. The Center's innovative, integrated treatment program is firmly rooted in both the newest neuroscience findings about the brain's ability to restructure itself, and the ancient medical sciences of many cultures, especially China's.

The staff at CIREN includes neurologists, neurosurgeons, physical therapists, Traditional Chinese Medicine practitioners, homeopaths.... Wait. Did you say homeopaths and neurosurgeons? I did. Cuban medical students learn principles of homeopathy, Chinese medicine, and herbal medicines from other traditions. At CIREN, you can expect both the latest in three-dimensional brain imaging and a course of Bach flower remedies to be part of your individualized plan. This plan is developed over the course of a full week of diagnostic tests of all kinds, interviews and consultations. Then they put you to work. For the next month, patients are in treatment of one sort or another for seven hours a day, five and a half days a week. The results, by all accounts, are astonishing.

Health care is free to all Cuban citizens. Cuba also sends doctors all over the world to treat and teach, and has developed a thriving health tourism industry. People from many countries come to Cuba to get top-notch medical treatment at a fraction of what it costs in their own countries. But a fraction of what this kind of intensive "restoration" program would cost in the US is still a lot of money. US citizens pay $20,000, not the $200,000 a co-patient of mine in Berkeley paid for roughly half the rehab hours CIREN provides, but we still can't afford it.

I am getting this treatment for free through the generosity of Cuban Revolution partly because a few key people know about my work as a radical writer, but mostly because my father is deeply loved and respected there. I called him up and told him he had to get over his reluctance to ask for favors. Together we crafted an email, sent it, and within days were told that the Minister of Public Health had instructed the Director of CIREN to provide me with a free course of treatment.

The Cubans don't ask for repayment of their generosity. No one will ever imply that I owe them anything. But I do. We all do. They are living proof that really excellent health care can be provided to an entire population for pennies on the dollar of what we spend here, when the primary commitment is to the wellbeing of people, not corporations. Because they dared to set up a society that rejected the whole premise of a profit-driven world, Cubans have paid a bitter price. For half a lifetime, the United States has tried to strangle their experiment in human based economics through a vicious trade embargo and blockade, upheld by a massive disinformation campaign aimed at persuading the people of the United States and the world that what's going on there is evil.

Every week I get Bowen bodywork treatments for injuries to my shoulder, the result of too many bad landings during seizures. Angie, my body worker, has heard of CIREN because she met an Argentinian woman at a training who had gone there to accompany a client. She asked so many questions about the treatment that they said, "Why don't we just train you?"

"How come they have such good medicine?" she wants to know.

I say their researchers can follow their hunches toward what works, without thinking about patentable product. That they aren't funded by drug companies. I say, "Doctors aren't privileged the way they are here, you don't do it to get rich. You do it for other reasons." I say they aren't bound to the bottom lines of HMOs. Frugality is important in a poor and blockaded nation, but the administrators of clinics and hospitals, the developers of health care priorities, are directed by their society to provide as much as possible, not as little.

"I guess they're not as bad as we've been told," she says. "Why do you just hear bad things about them?"

"Because rich, powerful corporations that want to own everything don't like it when people say no. It's because they said no."

12:30 pm The Luggage Center, Berkeley, CA

Without knowing the bulk of what I will carry, I am eyeballing duffle bags and suitcases for the load of medical supplies I hope to take with me. I keep asking my Cuban contacts if there are items I can bring, ways I can leap the blockade and smuggle them tidbits, for pleasure or necessity—but they won't tell me. Every one of them writes back, don't bring us anything. Sitting and talking with you is all the gift we need. Finally I ask my father about it. He says they don't want to take advantage of having US friends when their neighbors don't.

There is also the issue of visitors from a rich country, the same one that is causing so much suffering, dispensing bars of soap and getting to feel generous, when what Cubans need from us is political action and respect. My friend with decades of relationships there says it makes her furious when USers hand out chewing gum to Cuban children. She says, take gifts related to work. Blank CDs, flash drives, professional journals. My father says music and books, things we have because they are unique to our cultural life, not because we live in the crumbling center of an imperial economy.

I know part of my struggle is my difficulty in just accepting the great gift I'm being given. Being disabled and chronically ill for so long, and needing so much help from individuals, I am always trying to manage the balance of trade between my life and the lives of others, not wanting to overdraw my accounts.

2 pm Wheelchairs of Berkeley

I am here to have my wheelchair thoroughly checked and tuned for travel, to replace the leg support that bent when a guy on a work bike crashed into me, to get a new battery and learn how to disconnect the leads when I get on planes. There are two young men in the waiting room.

The white one in the power chair is conducting elaborate negotiations by cell phone with his father and his father's secretary and the receptionist and the insurance company. Fixing his chair will empty his bank account. Since his chair was bought out of pocket, the insurance may not cover repairs. Does he have a prescription for repairs? A flurry of faxing follows.

The Black man is a little older, and I can't tell whether his drooping face and unfocussed eyes are the result of weariness, illness or drug use—or possibly, given poverty, discouragement, and pain, all three.

His manual chair is literally held together with red plastic tape. The rim to the wheel, the seat to the frame. It looks like it will dump him in the street at any moment. The receptionist says the problem is he asked for a new chair instead of a replacement chair. He will have to fill out a new form and start the authorization process all over.

We sit, steeping in our frustration and boredom in the front of the store, like patients in a hospital emergency room. An hour after my appointment time I am called back into the repair alcove, where bolts are tightened, the charger tested, new leg supports ordered. When I come out an hour later, the two men are still there, waiting.

On the way home, I decide to stop by Herrick Hospital to see if M. is there. For nine months, with gaps while we waited for reauthorization, M was my physical therapist, working with sensitivity and ingenuity to help me deal with intense post-stroke pain that made touch unbearable, the weakness and swelling of my right foot and hand, the lack of coordination, and the need to either find new ways of doing things or have someone else do them. I find her behind the counter and tell her I've done it—I am actually leaving for Cuba in three weeks. Her face lights up as she comes to hug me. We talk for a while, and as I am leaving, as she wraps her arms all around me and kisses the top of my head, she says I deserve this.

I think of my friends with out of control seizures. The ones with MS and Parkinson's. About the people I love who have mysterious ailments they can't get diagnosed, because the tests have to be fought for, because the specialists rule, and no-one talks to anyone else, because some aspect of their being offends the gatekeeper. Like the sleep specialist I went to, who saw I was middle aged and female and kept asking me over and over if I was sure I wasn't just neurotic and what made me think I was epileptic? Like the dermatologist I went to because I had pale smooth patches of skin on my face, who told me I should bleach the rest to match, that it would make me beautiful. Like the ER doctor who kicked my transgendered friend out of the hospital with a fever of 104 degrees. M is right that I deserve the care I'm going to get. So do we all.

Havana Blog, 2009

May 30, 2009

We start the day at 6:30 AM, in a lovely accessible bed and breakfast in Cambridge, Mass, and by 7:30 are loading nine bags and two wheelchairs into a taxi for our Air Canada flight to Montreal. Our driver is a laid off hotel manager turned taxi driver, the fourth exiled Moroccan to help us on our journey. Cab drivers, nurse's aides, and airport employees can teach you all about globalization.

When we get to Air Canada's desk, they ask if we'd like to go on an earlier flight with a larger cargo bay for my power chair, so we take off for the 38-minute flight over New England. and spend the day at the Travel Lodge in Montreal, resting and looking for edible food. This time the cab driver is from Mauritania and proves unreliable, as does the porter who promises to meet us in ten minutes where we've checked our bags.

The result is that we get to Cubana late, and I have to fight with the Montreal based employees about whether my chair can go on the plane. One man tries to tell me it will have to stay in Montreal until I return. I just keep repeating that I need it, and eventually the man who actually has to fit things into the cargo hold shows up and figures out how to do it.

Then we have Canadian Customs. What freaks them out most is my possession of yogurt, "a creamy substance," and the also the screwdriver for disconnecting the wheelchair battery. They want a note that proves that it's medically necessary for me to eat. They need a supervisor to authorize the tools. The Cubana desk clerk has told us to run. Customs tells us to wait. Eventually, the top Cubana representative is found and authorizes tools and yogurt, and we're told the chair will probably make it, so we go on board.

By now it's been twelve hours of travel, and I'm exhausted to the point of nausea—too tired to enjoy reading, ready to arrive. A half-hour out from Havana everyone begins chattering, a sound track of happy excitement like a multitude of chirping sparrows. And then the lights of Havana are below us, and we land.

We stay in our seats, waiting for wheelchair service. I'm expecting it to take a while, but suddenly two men in guayaberas wearing tags from MINSAP, the Ministry of Public Health, appear on the plane, talk with the crew and come over to us, announcing they are here to help me to a manual chair while my power chair is unloaded. They will stay with me, they assure me, until I'm at the van.

At the bottom of the ramp is a smiling woman with a clipboard, looking amazingly fresh and relaxed given the late hour.

"Aurora?" She asks. When I say yes, she says she's Rosa from CIREN, here to welcome me. The MINSAP guys and a large male nurse from CIREN take the bags from Leah's hands and we go off to customs. Here the yogurt and tools don't interest anyone. It's the CPAP machine that needs explaining. Rosa tells me that the director has told her to take very good care of Sra. Aurora. When I mention that I'm from Puerto Rico she says, "We know." As we roll down the ramp into the airport, my eyes fill with tears. She asks what's wrong, and I say I'm happy. She says, "Estás emocionada?" Are you moved? Good. "Eso es bueno."

Outside, four Cuban men and Leah are trying to figure out how to fit all our luggage, plus all the people, into the small van. It's a complicated three dimensional puzzle involving a lot of hilarity, improbable suggestions and improvisation.

"Come on," Rosa says. "Let's go change your money," and we leave them to it.

When we get back to the van, people are eyeing Leah's slender build and proposing that she and Rosa share a seat, when the nurse says he's going to take the wheels off the manual chair, and stow them above the suitcases. The driver says doubtfully that it will be difficult. The nurse is scornful. If he can take the wheels off trucks, he can handle a wheelchair.

Sure enough, in two minutes we're all in, though the back doesn't latch and there are jokes about people running behind us picking up bits of our belongings. We drive through the tropical night to Neuro Villa, the complex that houses patients from two of CIREN's five clinics. In the pre-revolutionary 1950s this was a wealthy neighborhood, where, among the once stylish suburban houses, the bodies of tortured dissidents were dumped in the bushes. The weathered homes now house five to six patients, along with the support person each one of us has brought along to help with basic care.

We've been assigned one of the best rooms-— a small suite with a bedroom, a spacious living room and an immense bathroom with cement tile floor and fluorescent lights on the walls. Air-conditioned, thank God. Cuba in summer is no joke. And waiting there is Lula, the nurse on duty, radiating warmth and ready for a preliminary intake interview at 1 am. She says the on call doctor would have come by as well, but they decided to let us sleep. When he does come, the next morning, he asks repeatedly if we have any problems he can solve.

Lula says they're going to take good care of me. Over and over, everyone tells me I'm home, that I'm among family now, that I'll be cared for. Lula gets up to go. She smiles and turns out the light. "Estas en tu casa."

May 31, 2009

Awake at dawn. Bird song fills the air and I get up and go to the door to get my first glimpse of CIREN by daylight. There are trees everywhere: palms, banyans, almonds, flamboyanes, a small pomegranate, and lush, brightly colored shrubs. Our house has five patient bedrooms and a shared dining area. Lula has said to call her when I wake up, so she can introduce me to the other staff. Nurses work one day on and two days off, and the next nurse has just arrived. Lula also introduces me to the cook, and the woman who will be cleaning our rooms.

Right now there are only two other patients in our house— one Cuban and one Venezuelan. A Haitian woman will be coming with her son in a few days. Lula and the second nurse, Bárbara, look at my power chair and agree I won't be needing it except for the longest transfers. I say I'll use it to explore the neighborhood. In chorus they say: "Just at the beginning." Lula adds firmly, "You won't need it after that. You can count on giving it away or selling it."

I'm a little shocked. No nurse in a US hospital would say something like that. What with liability and the fear of offering "false hope, " every word about outcomes is cautiously framed. I try to explain this to Lula. She says, "I don't mind being wrong, and if I am it will be a pity, but I'm not. You'll see. We have a whole cemetery of canes and chairs."

Lula and Barbara and the cook confer about my allergies and decide I should eat from my supply of sardines until I speak with the dietitian. Trying to get me yogurt and the Cuban sweet potato known as boniato, before there's been paperwork, will involve "tramites," strings to pull and bureaucratic hoops to jump through. I dine on sardines and fresh tomatoes. Then Leah and I go for a walk to buy produce and explore. We end up getting ripe pineapple slices and cucumbers. For lunch, they've made me rice, grilled chicken, and a tomato and cucumber salad. It's delicious. I don't at all mind the prospect of daily chicken and rice.

The first co-patients we meet are Robney and his mother Teresa, here from Venezuela. Six years ago Robney was in a serious car accident, with a skull fracture and bleeding in his brain. He was in a coma for 18 days. Three years ago, when he first came here, he couldn't speak or walk. Last night at dinner he told us he'd walked 6.2 kilometers at the gym that afternoon.

"Paso por paso se llega a Roma," he tells us. Step by step you get to Rome. When we meet, he looks me over and says, "One month. In one month you'll be walking."

"Thank you. I hope so," I say, smiling.

"No," he says. "It's your decision. You have to work. We're the ones who do it."

They are finishing their second 28-day cycle.

"You've landed in the best there is," Teresa says.

Robney's speech is hesitant, as if he needs to search for words. I saw him earlier, walking slowly along the side of the street with a young woman. His right arm is in some kind of splint. They came here after he woke from his coma and got surgery. Now they're back for the long, slow rehab.

"This is thanks to our president Chavez," Teresa says. "He wrote it into the constitution that health is a right. They can't take it away from us now unless they have another coup and run off with the whole constitution." Under agreements between the Cuban and Venezuelan governments, Venezuelans come here with all expenses paid. Cuba exchanges medical care for oil.

June 2, 2009

It's dawn in Cuba, the beginning of my first full day of testing at the International Center for Neurological Restoration

Over lunch, Teresa tells us more about Robney's accident. It was music that brought him out of his coma, so he could travel here for brain surgery. It's his third visit. This time around he's been at CIREN for two months and has another month to go. From time to time he bursts into song, romantic Venezuelan love songs in a rich tenor voice. He is relearning to read, and then plans to study music.

Venezuelans make up the largest nationality of foreign patients at CIREN, which has seen 40,000 people from 84 countries since its establishment by Fidel Castro in 1989. 22,000 have been Cubans. We learn this at our new patients orientation, where we meet two more Venezuelans, including an indigenous man from Ciudad Bolivar, and an Angolan woman whose son can neither hear nor speak, an aftermath of malaria. She took him, she says, to a military hospital in Angola, and a Cuban doctor named Raúl told her to apply to CIREN.

The second Venezuelan, the talkative mother of a fifteen year old, says doctors in her country told her the girl would always use a catheter and never walk. But when Cuban doctors evaluated her, they said she didn't need the catheter and had an 80% chance of walking, so here she is. The woman also tells us about Carolina, whom the staff remember, a quadriplegic woman who was here for two years and now walks, using only a brace, from the knee down, on one leg.

Last night we received a visit from Maria Concha Morales, Mary Conchy, as she's called, a doctor and professor of traditional medicine at the Policlínico Plaza in Havana. She and her friend, a medical researcher, came to collect a suitcase of donated medicines and books. Within minutes she's read my pulse, working pressure points on my body, and teaching my helper Leah how to do Tuina massage on my back, until the skin can be easily lifted away from the muscles. She has also offered to set up Reiki training for us both, saying it's the most fundamental level of healing work because it draws on my own energy. It's an agreement with myself, not with an outside force. All the rest, the herbs, flowers, medicine, will work much better. Leah and I must become Reiki sisters. How's Sunday?

She also presses special points to relieve an attack of my sniffing tic, and arranges to put a complete alternative emergency medicine course on my flash drive. She lights up when she sees that we've brought her a 2006 Physician's Desk Reference. "¡Qué maravilla! Now, this is a gift!," she says. "For this," she says with a grin, "we'll teach you a course every week!" I ask her about chronic fatigue, how they treat it. For us, she says, chronic fatigue is from not wanting to be here and now. Epilepsy is wind in the liver. How do I sleep? Terribly, I say, and she says sleep is the most important neuro-restorative there is.

"We have to take care of that yesterday! Your closet full of pills won't do you any good without sleep." Slow deep breathing, the pressure points for insomnia and the back massage from Leah. That's the homework.

When I mention my power chair, how they tell me I won't be needing it, she asks me if I've read Deepak Chopra.

"You have to want this for yourself. You have to imagine it or you won't get it." I tell her I've done that for years.

"Yes," she says, up here— touching her forehead. "But you have to do it here—from your heart."

I tell her about Robney's long walk the day before, how it occurred to me for the first time, after hearing him, that I could hike again. I tell her about my favorite trail in Redwood Park, in the Oakland hills, and how much I love it, and she lit up.

Her visit has made me relax about all the allopathic medicine in store for me. The epileptologist who passed by yesterday seemed set on giving me drugs. He will be the head of my personal team of five or six practitioners. But after listening to my history, he seems willing to just recommend the meds without imposing them.

This morning I will have blood drawn for a whole range of tests, get an EEG, a neurophysiological evaluation, and a psychology evaluation. This kicks off a full week of tests. On Saturday they'll unveil my personalized plan.

Before I left Berkeley I decorated my wheelchair with my photograph, and brought a bag of rhinestones to glue on every available surface. After listening to Lula, I can't do it, and I'm removing the photo today. A year ago I wrote that my wheelchair was an exoskeleton. Yesterday it became a bridge that I will cross and leave behind.

June 3, 2009

The first day of testing started with an auditory exam that measures how long it takes sound to travel from my outer ear through the various stages to my brain, and a nerve test that measures the passage of sensation up my arm—the sensation is an electric pulse, unpleasant on the left side and painful on the right. Then the EEG, and home for lunch.

I tell Lula I've never had some of these tests, how everything in the US is measured out in the tiniest increments, how every single thing has to be justified. I end up telling her about the abusive ambulance crew that mistreated me so outrageously just before I left. She says she went to Chile once with a patient. She said they had everything, things Cuba lacks, but the nurses would give their patients medicine, and say maybe three words to them. "The most important part is this," she says, gesturing back and forth between us—"the human relationship."

She has asked me to bring the power chair to the test site because the clinic we're going to has big ramps and it will save her having to push me uphill.

"But don't identify with the chair," she says, "it doesn't belong to you. It's just borrowed." I tell her what I wrote about it being a bridge.

"Good," she says. "write it down." I tell her how much difference it made when I got it, and she says she understands that it played an important part in my life, but that was a stage, and it's over.

We also talk about shortages. The bathroom at the clinic has no toilet paper or soap. When I tell her, she shrugs, then goes and gets me a small piece of TP from an office. Later when I'm being amazed about all I'm getting, she says "But we lack a lot of things, almost everything." I say I know.

She says "Yes, but reading it is one thing. Now you're living it."

We talk about the intense alienation of the US, how a lot of the time people don't know their neighbors or make the kind of commitments to one another that are the fabric of life here. "We don't have things, but we have ganas—the will—and that goes a long way. In the US you have all kinds of things, but no ganas."

So Leah and I learn to use a hose instead of toilet paper and soak up the ganas everyone has to be of help to each other and to us.

June 4, 2009

After today's morning tests, Leah and I head out with Gabriel the taxi driver, to run some solidarity errands. First stop. ACLIFIM, the national office of the organization of people with physical disabilities, where we meet Ana, with whom I have corresponded. We're shown into a room whose walls are covered with gorgeous, brilliantly colored paintings, the work, Ana tells us, of a quadriplegic man who painted with a brush held in his teeth. Not knowing exactly where to start, I ask about disabled artists.

"Oh, yes," she says, "We have an annual festival. It begins at the local level, and then artists compete for places in the provincial, regional and national festivals. This year's event was just last month." I try to imagine government municipal, county, state, and national disabled artists' festivals in the US.

The Cuban constitution guarantees full equality to all people, so there is no equivalent to the ADA, no law specifically made to guarantee the legal rights of the disabled. ACLIFIM steps in to see to it that the existing policies are carried out. For example, every Cuban has the right to a free education all the way through graduate school, but there is still individual prejudice, which can create administrative barriers. ACLIFIM intervenes in such cases. They also do public education, working to bring popular consciousness into line with government policy.

Disabled people are guaranteed the right to work. Ana tells us there is zero unemployment for any disabled person who wants to work. If a disabled person trains in a particular field, and there is a place near them where that kind of work is done, they get a job there. If there is no job available, one will be created for them. This is when I cry.

Almost all disabled children are mainstreamed in school. There are two special ed schools, but these are seen as transitional programs, with as many children as are able moving into their local public schools. For children in other areas of the country, for whom the mainstream classroom will not work, a traveling teacher comes to the home to do instruction, but takes the child to the local school a couple of times a week to make friends and develop social skills.

I show Ana the materials I have brought from Axis Dance Company and Sins Invalid, whose work centers on disability and sexuality. She is thrilled, and starts talking about organizing an international disability and dance festival. They haven't ever invited foreigners before.

I ask her what are the biggest problems they face. Access, she tells me, is number one. Streets, buildings, transportation are not accessible, and though there are plans to change this, the blockade, with its resulting shortage of material goods, and overall economic impact, makes it very difficult. Cuba has a severe housing shortage, which, combined with the lack of accessible buildings, impacts disabled people especially hard. There is also a major shortage of wheelchairs, although two factories have just been built to start manufacturing them in Cuba.

Later in the day, as we roll along the Malecon, Havana's eight kilometer waterfront walkway, we pass one man and then another in old manual chairs. Both are missing legs. I'm in a folding manual chair which I brought in order to leave here, and I consider it pretty uncomfortable compared to the power chair. The first man stares openly at it and says "That's good!" I move closer so he can look, and he takes in every detail, stares after me when we move on. The second man cranes his neck, and a few minutes later we see him coming back in our direction to look again. I'm glad I'm not in the power chair. It would be like driving a Rolls down a muddy track where people struggle with mules. Much too much wealth. I'm glad I'm planning to leave the manual chair here, but I wish I could give it away thousands of times over.

Shortages are not what they were in 1993, the year I came with Global Exchange's Freedom to Travel trip, 175 USers defying the travel ban. At the height of the special period, there were almost no cars on the road, only a few hours a day of electrical power, and not enough food. Now there are urban farms everywhere, people look well fed and there is traffic, but none of the bathrooms have toilet paper or soap. I give one of the nurses an extra bottle of the hand sanitizer I brought, made from oil of thyme and oregano.

Next stop is CENESEX, the center for sex education. The building is undergoing massive renovations, so the woman who comes out, to find out what we want, meets us in the small outer reception area, with dust and tools all around. Magaly Gonzalez Jimenez is one of the specialists on staff. When she grasps that I'm there to give them things, not ask for them, she is delighted. When I tell her about Sins Invalid, she gets really excited.

"That's just what we're starting to work on," she says. "You can help us!"

There is going to be an international sexology conference in January and I should get people to come. And to write for their journal, Sexology and Society. The radio is on in the background and she says, that's one of our staff people. She turns it up so we can hear. The speaker is explaining that when a trans man is in a relationship with a woman, this is a heterosexual relationship.

Directed by Mariela Castro, daughter of Raul Castro and feminist pioneer Vilma Espín, CENESEX has pioneered trans liberation work in Cuba, as well as work on lesbian, gay and bisexual liberation, all of which comes under the heading of sexual diversity. In the entryway is a poster of two shaving brushes side by side. "Two of a kind can make a pair," it says. By the time we leave we are loaded down with educational materials, including a book on transexuals in Cuba, all of which will be invaluable for my writing.

"These are some of our three a.m. hallucinations," Magaly says, smiling. "Things we dream up."

They include pamphlets on STD/HIV prevention specifically written for different populations: adolescents, medical students, cross-dressing men known here as transvesti. We leave with an appointment to come back in July, and several copies of their journal.

On the way home we stop for more phone cards and a bottle of hot sauce, because after that first meal, the food has been dreadful. No one can tell me why there's no seasoning on the daily slab of greasy chicken. We also picked up some ripe tomatoes and limes. Tonight's chicken will be much more flavorful.

June 5, 2009

Day three. I've now had a series of tests to establish a baseline for my motor function, including a lot of measurements of my legs and arms—an intriguing combination of high and low tech. Also a dental check up, and a nearly two hour holistic medicine evaluation that begins with the doctor throwing his arms wide open and shouting, "Come give me a kiss!" He met my father at a scientific conference a few years ago. Tomorrow I'll have an MRI, some x-rays, and a psychiatric evaluation, which is always included for epileptics.

The dentist talked to me about my tooth grinding, explaining that there's a vicious cycle of tight jaw muscles and tooth grinding that can be interrupted by a combination of wearing a tooth guard to stop the signal to the brain created by contact between my teeth, and by practicing consciousness of the habit, and deciding to stop. She also recommended using a muscle relaxant at times of stress, to interrupt the cycle from the jaw-muscle end. So they'll be making me a mouth guard!

The holistic doctor talked about life lessons, how every circumstance offers opportunities to learn what we're supposed to—how to live.

"It isn't a matter of intensity—we should live as intensely as we are able to support. It's about balance. The sun is more intense than we can imagine. It lights up the whole solar system and supports all life, but it's in balance."

His perspective on Chronic Fatigue was fascinating. He said fatigue was a symptom not an illness, with many possible causes, and that it was dangerous to treat adrenal fatigue by itself, that often this involved stimulating the adrenals when the underlying strength to support it wasn't there, and this could make things much worse. He said I had excess liver chi constitutionally, which often leads to weak kidneys and pancreas, and that from his point of view the pancreas was the central issue.

My blood work shows somewhat elevated sugar, but he was speaking of the pancreas in all its functions— immune, endocrine, exocrine and digestive. Although his work is usually limited to supporting the neurological rehab, he said that in my case, for love of my father no doubt, he'll work with me to create a plan of action for the whole complex of other problems I have. Diabetes, he says, is associated with over-worry. That will be the emotional aspect of the work. For all of us, he tells me, it's about learning to live, learning the art of living in balance.

June 8, 2009

Well the hot sauce was a disaster because I broke out in hives, had to get a shot of Benadryl and was groggy for the rest of the day. That was Friday. On Saturday it happened again, this time with tomatoes. But with the help of homeopathic Apis, a remedy made from bee sting, I managed to avoid more than a small dose of antihistamines, and we were able to follow through on our plans for the day.

Vega is an electrical engineer who does a little work as a driver on the side, and my friend Karen has known him and his family for years. Silent at first, as he drives us across the city to the neighborhood of Santo Suarez, he opens up, and begins a running commentary on the neighborhoods we pass through, until we pull up in front of the home of my father's close friends and colleagues, Deisy and Miguel.

It's Miguel's mother's 90th birthday and there will be cake. Deisy's mother greets us with kisses and ushers us into a pleasant sitting room with high ceilings. Deisy emerges, her open face alight with pleasure. Leda will be here soon, she says. Deisy and Leda have known my parents for 33 years, working closely with my father throughout that time.

I tell them they are like cousins I've heard of all my life but never met. They beam at me, say that my father is like their father, too. I agree to share him, and they start telling stories from the various visits over the years. When I have explained my limited diet, Deisy proposes making me tostones and malanga—fried plantain and a boiled starchy root that I love. With the inevitable can of sardines I keep in my backpack, that will be a lovely meal. Deisy says I have to count on them more. When Leda and her husband Manolo arrive, we watch the short video message my father has sent, at my urging. They all melt at the sight and sound of him.

We talk about the health care system. CIREN is a specialist center, with nearly half the clientele coming from other countries, and is better resourced than some. There are hospitals from the

1940s still in operation. While the quality of the doctors and nurses is excellent across the board, that of support staff varies, and while some house patients three to a room, others have dormitory style rooms with up to 25.

Recently Deisy and Miguel's grandchild Beatriz suffered a terrible accident, colliding with her grandfather while he carried a pot of boiling water. At the burn center where they took her, there was another child with 2nd and 3rd degree burns over 60% of her body. Miguel says, "In any hospital anywhere, they'll tell you, you can't save a child burned like that, you ease the pain and let them go." The doctors debated what to do but fought hard for the little girl and were able to save her. But then, Miguel says, she'll need many operations, plastic surgeries, and where are the resources? Nevertheless, the doctors are amazing. While we're talking, young Beatriz, four years old, comes home, still bandaged over much of her head. She was in the hospital for quite a while and is not used to company yet.

I ask about the disparities between health care centers. It's complex, they say. There are hospitals that were here at the time of the Revolution, and many more were built in the 60s—-but we lack the resources to maintain them. The government wants to keep health care completely equitable, so they repair each one a little, when it would make more sense to pick a few strategically located ones and bring them up to the standard we want, and then do a few more the next year, and so on, instead of having them all be equally run down.

They tell me it's a problem born of overly centralized planning, bureaucracy, and an over-literal interpretation of equality. Then there are other issues that arose during the years of the Special Period. The Revolution raised people's aspirations, and then came a time of tremendous hardship, when their incomes couldn't begin to meet their goals. Some professionals left to work in other countries, in Latin America, Spain, the United States. The special period saw a resurgence of what Deisy calls anti-values, including the reappearance of prostitution, shady dealings connected to the double currency, opportunistic behaviors of various kinds, begging. They are excited about the prospects for some loosening up of over-regulation.

June 11. 2009

My physical therapist is Jorge, a young father of two, with eleven years experience and a passion for excellence. He's blown away by the DVD I lend him of Axis Dance Company—not just the beauty and power—what has him psyched is what it could mean for his patients, if they could learn to flip a fallen chair into the upright position the way dancer Rodney Bell does. He's thinking about paraplegics who don't leave their homes because of the impassible streets, who might brave the broken pavement if they knew they could right themselves from a fall. He takes it to the director, who misunderstands his excitement and thinks Axis could be a great cultural program for a disabled kid's school. She sees inspiration, not new rehab potential. So he takes it to one of the neurologists, starts talking it up to the other PTs.

"You have to work intelligently at things like this," he says, "plant little seeds."

Jorge and I talk, and work my body's weaknesses into strengths, for five hours a day. I hear about his four-year stint as a personal

PT in a mansion in Chile, with a millionaire family who had to be taught that they didn't own him. Which he apparently did on day one when he refused to work more than his contracted hours.

June 13, 2009

I've been too busy to write, and frustrated by the lack of access to my blog, and am running low on wifi time in the lobby of the incredibly, over-the-top hotel, Melia Havana, so just a quick update. I've had a lot more tests and more to come. They are determined to understand everything about my pain. The MRI machine, which was damaged when rainwater flooded the basement room it's in, is finally fixed, and I get my scan Monday morning, plus x-rays to check my spine for arthritis and other organic changes, and an ultrasound of my shoulder.

The physiatrist diagnosed fibromyalgia and prescribed magnetic and electrical treatments. I am SO well cared for here! I adore my PT, who gives the most amazing massages to ease pain in my pelvis and upper back. We alternate working out with weights, on a bike, doing leg lifts, etc., with heat lamp treatments. I started out on Tuesday walking 16 meters, and yesterday I did 50. I also started B12 shots for the neuropathy, which seem to help. Jorge says we'll reach our goal, to have me dancing again when I leave.

There's so much more to tell, but I have to protect my hands and not type too much. I'm having tech issues with my dictation program, which I'll try to crack tonight.

Today I sang Kalinka with the brain injured 18-year-old girl from the Ukraine who gets fine motor and cognitive therapy at the same time as me. It was a deeply lovely moment, as she often spaces out and is unresponsive.

Til soon.

June 16, 2009

Well fed turns out to be an exaggeration. At night, in the warm, damp air, I listen to the nurses talking about how they can't do birthday parties for their kids, how one mother made macaroni salad for her son, and then she invited people over and they ate up a whole bowl full, food for several days. Our new friends Myrtha and Alexis meet us in Old Havana and after some persuasion, agree to let us take them out for lunch at a reasonably priced place with delicious food— except that what's reasonable in CUCs, the "convertible" currency that has some relationship to foreign exchange and hard currency, turns out to be more than a month's salary in Moneda Nacional, the internal currency of Cuba.

My physical therapist makes about $20 a month in CUCs. A can of cooking oil costs $2.15. An electric fan is $35. The "canasta," a minimum monthly amount of food guaranteed to every Cuban, doesn't even begin to cover a month's worth of eating, so everyone contrives, and there isn't enough protein in most people's diets. The huge disparity between CUC prices and Moneda Nacional salaries is intimately related to the US blockade. I've gotten a variety of explanations about exactly how it all works, and look forward to meeting my friend Karen's neighbor who is an economist. It least part of it is an attempt by the Cuban government to manage their commitment to guarantee nutrition by subsidizing certain basic foods, and deal with the distorted trade relations created by imperial bullying, and get hold of hard currency. Then there's the immense extra cost of importing things the long way around, since any country shipping to the US can't also ship to Cuba without penalties. Adding three stops can triple the price.

Still, things are easier than in that terrible time following the break up of the Soviet Union called the Special Period. Jorge says his high school girlfriend's grouchy, counter-revolutionary father would always ask him, "What's so special about it?" Jorge was in his last year at a very rigorous science and technology high school when the Special Period started. He says it was like going to sleep with everything and waking up with nothing. A soda and a hamburger bun for lunch. Never enough to eat, and a devastating power shortage, with so many rolling blackouts people talked about "alumbrones," the moments when the lights were on, instead of the blackout "apagones."

There was a joke that from the air, Cuba looked like a Christmas tree; when the lights when off in one place, they went on in another. Jorge says you could hear the cries of protest down one street and rejoicing on another as the power came and went. Whole neighborhoods went out to the Malecon, by the ocean, just to sit and talk somewhere other than their hot and dark houses.

"So when did the not so special period begin?" I ask. '97 or '98, he says.

"So things got better then?" Jorge laughs.

"No, no, they STARTED to get better."

Food became more available as people were given unused lots to farm, and the lights went on for longer and longer.

Arsenio, the revolutionary philosopher who cares for the pool, is fierce on the subject.

"Someday history will know everything the Cuban people did to just stay alive, to feed ourselves and stay free."

His rage about the blockade is sharp and clear. Inhuman, criminal, savage, cruel—what possible reason could there be to do such a thing to a whole people? I say it's vengeance for your independence and the dangerous hope you represent.

"But they didn't do this to Viet Nam, or China, or Korea!"

Arsenio is eloquent on several dozen subjects at a time, passionate about the revolution, which he joined as an eleven-year-old literacy teacher in 1961. He says when I get rid of all this crap, (waving a hand at my wheelchair,) we're going to go run around, and, by the way, I'm looking really mamey today referring to a lush tropical fruit. He has the most beautiful, coppery biceps I've ever seen. He's the one who tells me the gym used to be the home of one of the Bacardi family daughters. The mature fruit trees around the track are the remains of her garden, and the swimming pool he cleans is shaped like a letter B.

Two days ago we bought a fan. Therese, the wealthy Haitian whose beloved son got a brain tumor while in college, and has travelled the world seeking help for him, has gotten one from a friend and set it up in the dining room. But the one we borrowed from the kitchen, so we could play dominoes after dinner, gives off a smell of burnt rubber after five minutes of use, and seems about to burst into flames. The nurses and pantristas, the women who heat up and serve the food brought over from the main kitchens, are visibly wilting.

So now our new fan lives in the kitchen by day, and by night we do our part for the current energy conservation campaign by using it, instead of putting on two air conditioners in order to sleep. It is really, really, really hot. Thick, humid air that sticks to the skin. I can sit absolutely still and watch sweat drip from my body until my clothes are drenched. Yet, somehow I don't mind. I have adapted better than I could have imagined.

I've lost five pounds since I got here, a combination of all that sweating, many hours a day of working out and a week of nothing but yogurt and pumpkin for breakfast. Jorge and one of the other PTs laugh and say it sounds like Special Period food! Now it's supplemented by Cuban sweet potato, malanga and plantain, which we bought while waiting for the official approval of my diet change, only to find that Chinita, the pantrista, had also picked some up for me. But the best part is the garlic we got on Sunday at the public market! Now either Leah or Chinita fries up the boiled starches of the day with a good handful of chopped garlic and we share it with our Venezuelan friends, whose money has long since run out. Even the pumpkin tastes delicious.

Today was the second day of electrical and magnetic treatments, and the result has been amazing. My pain levels have dropped dramatically, and I'm able to walk much farther. The exercises that made my feet go icy and aching on Monday morning have become easy, and I can feel the fibers of my muscles growing strong. Jorge watches closely and announces that tomorrow we'll be adding more weights to every exercise. We have some catching up to do, since the first week, because of my pain, we worked well below the normal level. I'm lifting 33 lbs. with my stroke foot, and forty-something with the uninjured one. The goal is to push 20% above my own body weight. I ask when I'll get to use the walking machine. He says, when I can walk all the way around the track several times. Not if. When. Tomorrow we'll begin exercises to strengthen my back and ankles.

Today I also had laser acupuncture and learned a new, deliciously simple meditation technique. Carlos Manuel says I need to realign myself with natural cycles, rise early, work by day, go to sleep at night. Next week he'll inspect my supplements and hopefully thin them way down. And in between all the other healing activities, I had an ultrasound of my shoulder, done by a doctor, who showed me exactly what he was seeing—a chunk of missing cartilage where I repeatedly landed, hard, during seizures. But no inflammation, so we can start working my shoulder as well.

"Good," says Jenny, the "defectologa."

"I know he said ice, but what do you think about using heat?"

I'm all for it, in spite of the external temperatures. The heat lamps are marvelous, even if they're literally held together with silly putty and propped up with children's blocks.

I spend much of my time in defectology stringing beads, putting nuts on bolts, pegs in holes, and colored tiles into patterns I must memorize. Every day, right about the time my afternoon session starts, a handful of children in maroon and white school uniforms spills through the walkways and into the rooms where their parents work. They go to school two blocks away, and come here when it lets out.

They climb on the equipment, ask patients all about their rehab, clamber onto their parents' laps and generally make themselves comfortable. A five year old asks me how old I am. I tell her I'm 55. Her eyes widen. "You must be very long!" Yes, I tell her solemnly that I am. She peers under the table to check out my legs. Later she shows up in the gym and climbs onto a mysterious piece of equipment with a padded bolster she can swing on. Jorge patiently adjusts it to her height so she can play in safety, and then gives me my next instructions: OK, now do three sets of twelve with the right leg, and I press my calf onto the padded metal, take a deep breath and push.

June 25, 2009

This week the hardships, the logistical hassles and scarcities that are part of Cuban life have been a big part of ours. A week ago I flushed the toilet and sewage came bubbling up through the shower drain. The septic tank for the building is full, and our bathroom is closest to it, but there's only one sewage removal truck for the entire city of Havana, and it's sent according to priorities that are decided in some department somewhere. As my therapist Jorge says, "The situation is being analyzed."

First the authorities insist on moving us to a new room— and relocate all my things while I'm in therapy. But the new room is moldy, and so is each of the other available rooms. Eventually we're moved back and we use the bathroom at the other end of the building, in a room that's unoccupied because the air conditioning is broken.

Secretly, we use a bucket at night and empty it when no one who cares might be around. We're all praying it takes longer to fix the air conditioning than it does to get the truck to come. If a patient is put into that room, we have no bathroom and will have to be put somewhere else, though no one knows where. The roughest part was when we both got diarrhea and nausea, a regular summer occurrence around here, and had to use the bathroom a lot. We were given "sales" an electrolyte mix to prevent dehydration, and my Ukrainian friend slipped me a marvelous anti-diarrheal drug she brought from the Ukraine to Portugal and carries with her everywhere.

The Internet access that's on site was closed for ten days, since someone stole $50 CUC in cash in a pre-dawn break-in. This has meant getting a cab to go to the hotel Melia Habana to use the wifi in the lobby, which also costs more than access here. We had an arrangement with Vega, who drives us for about half the cost of a regular taxi, but his mother's been in the hospital, so he's been unavailable. She just got sent home because the hospital where she was is clearing out everyone they can in preparation for swine flu cases. There are 34 as of today, double the number of a few days ago.

Telephone access has also been frustrating. The only phone that works right now is the one inside the gymnasium complex, which is only open 8-6. Therapy is 8:30 – 5:30. I try to squeeze in calls at lunch or before therapy, but generally the times I'm free, people are on their way to work or on lunch break, and they get home after 6. If we could get hold of a Moneda Nacional Tarjeta Propia, a national calling card, we could call from a phone across the street that's always accessible, but no one can get the cards. Someone said they don't make them anymore. Someone else said she's been trying to get one from a friend at the phone company, but no luck. Those who already have them can recharge them, but whatever the real situation is, we don't have one and aren't likely to. The phone in our room could be hooked up—but it would take time, and cost 50 cents a minute for local calls. So we leave messages asking people to call, and hope they do it when we're in.

Tonight was a bonanza night. My parents called from Boston, and so did Leah's sweetie from California. It's amazing to hear the voices of our very own closest people!

This morning I walked 1300 meters! People have been congratulating me for the last several days, seeing me walk to therapy in the morning. The man who tends the Internet cafe came running out after us calling "Senora!" When I turned he said, "You're walking! That's wonderful!" He was beaming all over.

But then during weight lifting something went wrong, and I couldn't use my right foot at all: searing pain on the outside of my heel. We must have pushed it a little too much. This morning in rounds the doctor told the defectologist not to add weights to my arm exercises, because what with the allergic reactions and inflammatory pain, I clearly have some sort of autoimmune condition, even if they don't yet know what it is. Weights could make the pain worse. I think that's what happened with my foot. Very discouraging, going into the final week. I'm trying to figure out how to speed up the process of asking for a little more time here, if it turns out to be necessary.

I haven't mentioned my visit to the psychiatrist for my evaluation. I loved her! She asked intelligent questions, and when I told her I tend to be reactive and anxious she said calmly, "Yes, most epileptics are." She openly asked the nurse, right in front of me, if there were any questions about whether my seizures were psychogenic, asked me about any major traumas, told me I had good personal resources, that she'd like to help me finish getting over my terrible divorce, and generally reduce anxiety, and then, after warning me to stay away from psychiatric drugs ("They're really bad for you,") prescribed Bach flower remedies!

It's strange contemplating not eating dinner with Robney and Pajaro every night, not seeing the Ukrainian girl Anna and her mother every day, not spending most of my waking hours working out in the gym with the international crew of people who cheer each other on.

I came back to my room early, put ice on my foot, and turned on the TV, which is how I got to watch live as the Honduran people took to the streets to stop an attempted coup today. President Zelaya, yet another good Latin American president, has brought Honduras into ALBA, an organization of progressive Latin American countries working to build economic and political independence for the region. Following the examples of Venezuela and Bolivia, the Honduran people have been calling for a constituent assembly, so they can make constitutional changes that will allow for full popular participation in reshaping the country's future.

Honduras has been a strategic base of operations for the far right in Central America, and the oligarchy and parts of the military are up in arms. This Sunday there is a plebiscite about whether to put the constituent assembly onto the ballot in November. The military was in charge of getting the voting materials distributed to municipalities, and refused to do so. Congressional leaders called the vote unconstitutional and tried to block it. Zelaya announced an attempted coup, and people hit the streets by the thousands, in pouring rain, demanding that the military comply.

During the live coverage, Telesur, the multinational left news network based in Venezuela, ran people's text messages across the bottom of the screen. Most were messages of support, telling the Honduran people not to give up, that Venezuela was behind them, that we're all in this together, that they just had to say the word and Venezuelans would show up in Tegucigalpa. By late afternoon the head of the air force had sent word that the ballots would be delivered, and the people in the streets unloaded them, while brigades of volunteers got them to the municipal centers for distribution. The Minister of Defense has resigned, and a member of government whose title I don't know how to translate has said the armed forces will obey the law.

Although the struggles for true democracy and independence from US corporate control in Latin America represent some of the most hopeful news on the planet, the big transnational networks kept their gaze firmly fixed on the death of Michael Jackson. Yesterday we watched a series of programs about the five Cuban political prisoners held in the US, full of outraged responses to the US Supreme Court's refusal to hear their case. It was very powerful and moving. In between programs we watch "ads" about the importance of art, the building of energy independence in Latin America and the Caribbean, the importance of education for Latin America's children, and announcements of amazing shows we can't watch because they're on while I'm in the gym. I don't know how I'll stand being cut off from socialist television!

Saturday we head for the countryside with our "cousin" Leda and her husband Manolo. Sunday we've organized a shopping trip for vegetables in El Vedado with our Ukrainian friend, a delightful new Angolan neighbor, and an obnoxious Portuguese man I'm hoping we can ditch, since all he does is complain. In the late afternoon we'll go visit Alexis and Myrtha, and take Alexis some ink cartridges for the pen I gave him. He's a wonderful artist, completing a graphic novel of one of José Martí's books for children, all done in ball point pen. When I give him my fountain pen, his eyes fill with tears.

I've just been encouraged by the staff to apply for another month of treatment!

July 1, 2009

Today I met Conchita Campa, director of the Carlos Finlay Institute, which developed Cuba's meningitis vaccine. She is one of two women in the politburo, a passionate advocate of natural medicine, and a friend of my father's. She came to fetch me at CIREN in order to bring me to the Institute, where she arranged for me to eat in their macrobiotic cafeteria. After weeks of atrocious food at CIREN, slabs of over-cooked, greasy turkey, white rice and starchy roots twice a day, every cell in my body sang halleluyah as I savored their brown rice pilaf, pickled radishes, steamed green beans, and lentils.

Conchita has arranged for Leah and I to get all our meals there for the rest of our stay in Cuba! Every day at lunchtime the cooks will pack up dinner and breakfast for us. As I sat sipping bancha tea, one of them came out with a big bag of rice cakes for me to take home!

Conchita is warm, bubbly, full of enthusiasm for her work of promoting natural medicine, though her day job is still inventing vaccines. She has, she says, the complete flower remedy collections from California, Australia and her favorite, Chile, as well as Bach's original 38. She will arrange for me to see their nutritionist, and a famous homeopath.

She asks what I do and I tell her I'm a writer. I say I'd love to connect with other writers, get to read my work. "I'll call the Minister of Culture," she says. I tell her I'd love to spend some time in Cuba writing.

"All things can be arranged," she says, smiling. And then, "Wait a minute!"

She zooms out and returns with a man who directs a cultural foundation. He also eats here every day, and his work is to support the arts. He promises to arrange for me to see Nancy Morejon, the national poet laureate, and connect with people at Casa de las Americas, where a new program for US Latina/o writers and artists has just been launched. Also a network of women writers. And set me up to do a reading.

I mention that my brother is a visual artist. "Let's do an exhibit," he exclaims. I say I only have a few of his posters with me.

"No matter. Have him send digital images. We'll put up some posters and project the images and you can read. It'll be great!"

He says he'll get back to me tomorrow. After weeks of trying to grab minutes out of rehab time to access a phone, trying in vain to reach people whose names I've been given, suddenly I'm hooked up. Conchita and I adore each other from the first phone call. She says her family is full of Auroras, so I'll fit right in, and what's my sign. I decide she will get one of Ricardo's posters of Marx meditating, with the slogan "Synthesis." She loves it.

Today I also speak with Rosita from International Relations, who tells me I have to be like Cubans, do a little bit every day to resolve complicated logistical problems, and not let myself get stressed. My sacrum has been out for a few days and once again I can't do my exercises. My foot is better, though, so I walk a lot. Jorge says I have to strengthen my back muscles. Conchita says once I start eating well, the inflammation will go away. Tomorrow I should hear back from the Ministry of Public Health about my second cycle of treatment. If all goes well I'll take a week off before starting round two. A week for visiting Cenesex, ACLIFIM, Casa de las Americas and the new friends we've made.

Besides the stress of unresolved housing, food and authorization issues, this week has been all about the coup in Honduras and the ongoing evidence that Latin America and the Caribbean are in a new stage of history, where thugs can no longer get away with kidnapping elected presidents and terrorizing their own people into submission. Cuban TV and Telesur have been carrying detailed coverage almost continually: the proclamations of the

OAS, the ALBA nations, the Central American nations, the Rio countries, the UN, all condemning the coup, refusing recognition to the de facto regime, withdrawing ambassadors, cutting off trade. The OAS has given the golpistas 72 hours to step down. Zelaya has declared he will return at that time, accompanied by the secretary general of the UN, the president of the OAS and several presidents of Latin American countries.

In place of ads for useless and toxic products, we see photomontages of the right wing Honduran congress voting for one of their own to replace Zelaya, of Hondurans in the streets, of heads of state condemning this attempt to turn back history and restore the evil days of dictatorships and death squads. We also continue to get live reports from all over Honduras via cell phone. Somehow Telesur and Cuban national TV have the phone numbers of dozens of resistance leaders.

Today I saw Pedro, who came from Venezuela with his wife one day before I arrived. We were on the same buses to get our tests during the first week. He has Parkinson's, and when I first saw him, I couldn't understand anything he said, he walked with a shuffling gait, and he shook constantly. I sat with his wife on a park bench today, watching him stride around the track, catch and throw balls, and speak clearly, with no tremor at all! They will be leaving soon, but will return for one month a year, until the center modeled on CIREN opens in Venezuela.

Right now I'm deliciously tired, sitting in front of a fan, getting ready to go send emails. Then we'll come home to our take-out macrobiotic dinner and go to bed early.

July 5, 2009

Late afternoon, with heavy rain. Everyone within hearing is tuned into Mesa Redonda, the national political commentary program, which is having all day special coverage as we await President Manuel Zelaya's arrival in Tegucigalpa, expected within the next half hour. In recent days the weather has felt like being hit on the head with a hot frying pan, a physical burden of heat and light pressing down on us.

The combination of high temperatures and rain has unleashed the usual seasonal flu, and several therapists have been out sick with fevers and diarrhea. Two of our friends were quarantined in a neighborhood that had a couple of cases of swine flu. Telesur is on in the background as we wait for events that all of Latin America is watching closely—golpistas, as well as the people who have been building what is being called our second independence.

We just saw Honduran soldiers open fire on a crowd of demonstrators. The people had pushed through, as they thought, into the airport, but it turned out to be an ambush. Zelaya's plane is 20 minutes out. The reports are coming in via satellite cell phones. Chavez has just said the dignity of the Americas is on that plane. As I write it's being announced that two people have been killed. We're seeing the crowds, the teargas, hearing the shots and shouting via cell phones and the TeleSur reporters' cameras, which get interrupted as they move around and sometimes lose their signals.

Telesur reporters are talking with Zelaya on his plane, telling him what's happening on the ground, and transmitting his messages to the people, which those who can get Cuban radio, or watch Telesur online, can hear and pass on to others. I'm sitting here with tears running down my face, typing. Zelaya continues to talk about reason and peace and the rights of the people, in the face of barbarism and violence. He says to the soldiers, "In the name of God, in the name of the people, don't take part in a massacre."

The national police chief has just said he's withdrawing his forces from the airport, and is holding the army responsible for the shootings. One of the dead was a 16-year-old boy. The shots came from army snipers on rooftops.

People are uploading video from their cell phones onto the Internet, which Cuban TV is monitoring and broadcasting. There are also independent radio broadcasts via Internet.

The army has parked vehicles on the runway so that the plane can't land—and the air force is threatening to intercept it if they don't leave—to shoot down a plane carrying a head of state and the Secretary General of the UN.

For tense minutes Leah and I sit holding hands, watching Zelaya's plane circle, soldiers massed on the airfield, lying down in combat positions with their guns at the ready, the trucks positioning themselves on the runway. Zelaya is on the phone again, saying what he sees below him, saying that the pilot is telling him they can't land without risking a crash. He says if he had a parachute he'd jump. The reporter updates him. She tells him that when his plane came into sight, the people burst into cheers. He says they'll try again tomorrow and the next day and the next, until they find a way to get him back into the country.

Minutes later: Zelaya's plane has turned away. Now it's Hugo Chavez on the phone saying that at one point he and Zelaya and Fidel and Daniel Ortega were all on the phone together. He calls on the soldiers of Honduras to stand down, not to stain themselves with their own people's blood, and also talks about class struggle in the hemisphere—how the people of Latin America will not allow the military, representing the oligarchies, to retake the continent, that what happens now is about the future of our children and grandchildren. He says the yanqui empire is responsible for this coup— not Obama himself, he says, but Obama is a prisoner of the empire.

What a high adrenaline day! Chavez says the pilots managed to outwit the Honduran air force and approach by an unexpected route, so that they were able to circle the airport. The army trucks had to scurry to get out onto the runway and block them.

By the time you see this blog, most of this will be old news, though I don't know how much of the detail you'll get in the US. What's so intensely powerful, so different for me, is that I'm watching revolutionary media, commentators who don't serve any corporate masters, who belong heart and soul to the liberation projects unfolding in our Americas. It's immediate, unmanicured, and incredibly courageous. Telesur reporters, already kidnapped once by the gorilas, are back on the ground, reporting from within the range of the soldiers' guns, broadcasting via different technologies minute to minute as things change— sometimes voice only, via cellphone, sometimes live footage via satellite, sometimes via internet.

As soon as the coup happened and we knew there was a news blackout, Radio Havana boosted its signal strength toward Honduras, knowing that with the Honduran networks broadcasting cartoons, Hondurans would have to rely on outside radio broadcasts to find out what was happening. Honduran students in Cuba call their relatives and friends, report what they hear to Cuban TV and then it's broadcast back to Honduras. Zelaya and Chavez are both frequently on the phone with the Telesur crews. Cuban television journalists are getting phone reports from leaders of the popular movements all over Honduras, with minute-to-minute updates.

Sometimes the people on the phones are running as they talk. They send messages to their people in other places. Everyone insists on non-violence. In between the live reports, including bits of cellphone video from marchers, there are commentaries on the distorted coverage by CNN, and statements by important Latin American political and cultural figures. They talk about the School of the Americas, the school for golpistas. About the attempted coups in Venezuela and Bolivia.

One of the remarkable things is how the demonstrators themselves, as well as Chavez and Zelaya, keep saying to the soldiers, "You belong to the people, don't shoot them, don't attack your own families, your own future, reconsider, your job is to defend your people, not harm them. Join us!" Zelaya says, "I forgive you, but history will not."

CNN continues to support the de facto government, which they recognize, although no government in the world does, broadcasting Micheletti's claim that not a drop of Honduran blood has been spilled, but I saw the blood.

Now Zelaya has retreated, and soon we hear that he's in Managua. He repeats that his place is among his people, supporting their struggle to defend their democracy. His wife,

Xiomara Castro, has come out of the safe hiding place where she's been sheltered, to stand among the leaders at the front of the demonstrations. When she heard of the death of that sixteen year old boy, she said she couldn't stay hidden anymore. If that boy's mother had the courage to take to the streets, than so would she.

The overwhelming emotion I feel is of being where I belong, a part of my continent, which is the most hopeful place on earth at this moment in history. No one here is confused about what this battle is about. People are highly educated, and well informed, and radical, and everyone knows that this is the war of the rich against the poor, the savage rebellion of the elites against a government that dared to impose a minimum wage, provide school lunches, lower costs for farmers, and worst of all, at the request of its citizens, to put a revision of the constitution on the table that would allow the people of Honduras to participate in real ways in the running of their country.

The people who brought about this coup want to turn back the clock. From one end of the continent to the other, people have said no, so loudly and forcefully that even the United States has had to publicly denounce the de facto thugs. Cubans, who have been under attack for fifty years, understand very well that, as people all over Latin America have been saying all week, "Today we are all Hondurans."

August 15, 2009

My last visit with the psychiatrist. I tell her I'm afraid of the return to isolation. "I don't know how to explain to you, " I say, "what life is like in the States, how different it is from this country, where you have each other, where no one is left alone."

She answers, "I know. I've traveled. I've been to your country. It's a very hard place."

This is her parting prescription for me. I must increase the levels of solidarity in my life. "Find people who share your values, do important work together, and have fun doing it."

These words, and the bag of organically grown Cuban turmeric for my liver, courtesy of Conchita's friend, are what I hold close to me as I begin to pack.

The very last day, I turn to Jorge, and all the patients and therapists in the big therapy gym and say, "Watch!" Then I dance, just as I promised before believing, all the way around the room.

Shock

October 13, 2009

Coming back to capitalism is like walking into a brick wall. It's like being hurled into the middle ages. Like returning from the future to a place where everyone thinks it was just a dream you had, and you say, "No really, I was in a country without advertising, where all the doctors are free, and anyone who wants to can go to graduate school without going into debt, where people say 'we' a lot more than they say 'I,'" and you realize you're talking in a language no-one understands.

Coming back to capitalism after three months out from under is like walking into a horror movie. In this country, my neighbor can spray pesticides in his back yard and even if it gives me seizures, his right to private property overrules my right to health, and the worst thing is that it seems self-evident to him that it should be so. In this country my last ambulance ride costs twice as much as my rent.

Many years ago I heard an activist from another country, somewhere with dictators and soldiers in the streets, say that in the U.S. everyone lived in a fog of confusion, that they couldn't see reality. It gave her the creeps. She would much rather, she said, be in her own country, where people knew what they were fighting for and against. And that was 25 years ago. Late stage capitalism has eroded people's humanity, has trashed the quality of people's lives so much that we've become accustomed to living in hell. People in Cuba spoke to me with such compassion about USers. They said, "We know how much the people of the US must suffer. Is it true," they would ask, barely willing to believe such a thing, "that people don't know their neighbors? I heard that no one meets your eye when you walk down the street. Is it really like that?"

The first thing I saw when I passed through customs in Montreal, when I set foot on virtual US soil, was a dazzling array of merchandise, literally blinding. I couldn't see a way through, because of all the gleaming glass and precious metal, the duty free jewelry, perfume, alcohol, clothing, all lit by spotlights, all reflecting back and forth in a dizzying shrine to consumerism.

It had taken me 24 hours to get through the ordeal of Air Canada's horrific policies and attitudes about disabled travelers, and only three minutes to say, "I just came from Cuba," and be nodded through by an unruffled US customs agent.

I'm back in the land where people defend their right not to help you, where an airline agent was actually reprimanded for picking up my water bottle when I dropped it. "She's determined to show she can travel without an attendant, so she doesn't get any help," her supervisor snarled.

Fast forward, please, past those excruciating hours, trying to get on one flight after another, because in spite of the fact that I was walking up and down in front of them, the head of customer relations said he couldn't let me on a plane without a doctor's letter documenting that I could walk. So since it was a Sunday, I had my father track down a doctor friend who has never laid eyes on me, to certify in writing that I could fly for an hour and a half unsupervised.

Fast forward to the bed and breakfast in Cambridge, where delighted employees take in my wheelchairless state and rejoice with me. Then my close friend Freda and I walk to Whole Foods. Faced with what now looks like an obscene overabundance of food, shelves packed to the point of explosion with trivial, expensive, individually wrapped snacks, the towering piles of produce, much of which will be thrown away, I feel sick, and dizzy and start sobbing right there in the aisle. I have to leave Freda to pay, and go stand in the street to get air, because it took Daysi three days to find chicken liver for the special meal she made us, that cost all three days' salary, and we saw yogurt once at the grocery store, one glorious day, and then the case was ever after sparsely stocked with beer, and sometimes you have to go to four or five different stands to get an avocado, if you're lucky and when I brought pizza for my farewell party at CIREN, the therapists fell on it like starving piranhas, and forget toilet paper. I am so angry and grief stricken at the same time. I am filled with loathing for the blockade.

It's been over a month now and I am slowly growing a thicker skin, adapting to our particular brand of starvation, the lack of human connection, of ganas. I listen to the voice of my Cuban therapist saying "no te dejes llevar," don't let yourself be carried away, and I try not to lose my balance in the face of my neighbor's absolute determination to have his house be his castle, and the hell with me and my body; in the face of the cynical pretense of health care reform; in the face of staggering medical bills and institutionalized indifference.

This is why I haven't posted on my blog. This is why I haven't written my cascade of articles yet. I've been in shock, trying to learn to breathe clouds of pollution again when my lungs had gotten used to inhaling the oxygen rich air of solidarity.

Today I Ran

Today I ran half a block to catch a bus. Eight months ago I was in a wheelchair, unable to walk more than 30 feet, slowly and with pain. In May of 2007 I had a stroke that left my right side weak, and plagued with excruciating nerve pain and circulation problems. It took three months to get approval for physical therapy from my US insurance company, and what I was given was short, once a week sessions, with long administrative gaps for a grand total of 20 visits, after which I got 50% of the cost of a power wheelchair and my case was closed.

My doctors and physical therapists were as trapped by the corporate medical system as I was. I had an excellent PT who, knowing she could do little to strengthen my muscles in the time allowed her, focused on reducing my pain and teaching me coping strategies. At the end of our time together, her goal for me was that I be able to ride the wheelchair to a local store and then park it and be able to move around the small shop on my feet.

But after the thrill of leaving my house on my own wore off, I wasn't content with my limited recovery. I knew a little about Cuban medicine and had a friend who'd been successfully treated in Cuba for spinal cord injury after her US insurance ran out. My father is a scientist who has worked with Cuban scientists for 45 years. Through one of the organizations he works with he asked for help for me, and I was offered a free course of treatment, which ended up lasting two months.

From the moment of my arrival, the difference between the two medical systems was profoundly evident.

For the first week I underwent a battery of tests and examinations. Some were standard tests I'd had before, but no one had ever done nerve conduction tests of my hands and feet, or looked for a neurological basis for my hearing loss. I also had intake interviews with a psychologist and a psychiatrist, and with a holistic medicine doctor. Based on the information gathered, a team was assembled to oversee my care.

I lived in a house, on a street of similar houses, each with 4-6 patients and their caregivers, and a resident nurse. Doctors were on call and very accessible. When I came down with the flu, an MD was at my door in five minutes. My neurologist was always clearly up to date on my daily progress. He would stop me in the street to ask how things were going.

For close to 40 hours a week, for eight weeks, I did "restoration" work 4 to 5 hours a day with my physical therapist, working my legs, feet and back, 2 hours with the "defectologist" working with my hands and arms and doing a little cognitive therapy, highly effective daily treatments with electrical current and magnetic fields for nerve pain, hydrotherapy for back pain, and twice weekly sessions with the holistic doctor who did acupuncture and other treatments.

So how was this different from an intensive physical therapy program in the States?

> 1. It didn't cost hundreds of thousands of dollars. While in my case it was free, other international visitors paid, depending on what country they were

from, between zero, in the case of Venezuelans whose government has an oil for medicine treaty with Cuba, to $20,000 for Europeans. The young woman I met during my treatments in Berkeley, signed up for their version of intensive care, two hours a day of physical therapy for two months, without any of the array of other therapies I got, and her parents had to sell their home to pay for it.

2.   The absence of a profit motive is felt throughout the Cuban health care system. No one recommends expensive, useless procedures or drugs. No one makes more money if I spend more. There's no pharmaceutical lobby setting policy or controlling research. So the orientation of doctors is to get the best results with the minimum of intervention. When my helper and I got a stomach flu, we were given electrolytes, not anti-diarrhea medication. My neurologist proposed ice packs instead of ibuprofen, telling me, "It's really not very good for you." The psychiatrist wrote out a scrip for Bach Flower Remedies and warned me away from anti-depressants.

3.   Because there's no market competition between approaches to healing, and no long-standing medical monopolies, there's a high degree of respect for practitioners of traditional medicine. The neurologist listens to the homeopath, the PT recommends acupuncture, Chinese medicine and homeopathy are part of standard medical training, and the director of the Finlay Institute, the country's premiere research institute for developing vaccines, supervised the successful homeopathic immunization of five million

people in 2008, and promotes a macrobiotic diet through workshops and a special cafeteria, where I was able to arrange to get my meals. I also had several appointments with a respected doctor of natural medicine who consults at a provincial oncology hospital. The first visit, which was a house call, included osteopathic treatment, homeopathic medicine for brain injury and a prescription for turmeric, which is known to scour plaque from blood vessels. This means it's relatively easy to develop an integrated approach to any individual case.

4. Both the psychologist and the psychiatrist operated from a model of easygoing self-acceptance, rather than trying to "fix" me toward an unreal model of perfect happiness. The psychiatrist cheerfully told me I was unbalanced, that small things knock me farther off center than most people. "You just have to practice not letting yourself get carried away. When you're knocked off-center, climb back on," she said. The psychologist told me, "OK, so you're reactive and sensitive. Everyone has their struggles and that's yours. Mine is that I'm slow," and talked with me about strategies for minimizing the impact of those struggles on my daily life.

5. Because malpractice suits are not a part of medical life in Cuba, on the one hand, no one recommends unnecessary testing as a form of self-defense for the doctor, and on the other, medical professionals are freer to try things. A former colleague of my therapist's who now practices in Florida, writes frustrated letters about how little he dares to experiment with his patients. At

CIREN, such experimentation has led to the successful treatment of patients with ataxia using ozone therapy. When I asked my PT what happens if his treatment causes an injury, he looked puzzled. "We treat it of course, and then try something different." Carelessness is addressed within the workplace, where no one works in isolation, and in the absence of personal profit for doctoring, there's no motive for promoting ineffective or harmful practices.

6. The absence of malpractice as a perpetual threat has another profound effect. Medical professionals are lavish with physical affection. No one expects to be charged with sexual harassment for hugging a patient, so they do, often. Hugs and kisses, caressing touches on the arm, ruffling of hair—loving touch is deeply integrated into human relations at CIREN.

7. In U.S. hospitals, confidentiality and privacy are seen as important values, and contact between patients is often actively discouraged. As a patient, I've accepted confidentiality as a substitute for respect; given how badly I've been treated in the U.S. medical system, my instinct is to keep as much control as possible over who has information about me, since my expectation is that it may be easily used against me in some way. At CIREN, patients work together in an open gym and therapists discuss their cases in public. Developing a sense of solidarity, of group effort, is much more highly valued than keeping the details of our physical struggles secret. We watched each other's daily progress, heard about the cases of incoming patients, learned about the specific catastrophes that

had landed each of us there, and formed lasting bonds of mutual support. The grueling work of recovery was made immeasurably easier by our laughing, crying and sweating together.

8. This atmosphere of mutual support was also startlingly evident in the relations between staff members. Some of the therapists' children attended a school near the clinic, and often came to the gyms after school, where they were welcomed warmly, allowed to play on unused equipment, and exchanged friendly greetings with patients.

On several occasions the therapist who worked with my hand, simultaneously coached a colleague's daughter for her upcoming history exam. When one person had a family emergency, the whole group immediately divided up support tasks. The sense of life as a collective project we're all in together pervades Cuban life in ways that are both obvious and subtle. As a US visitor, accustomed to the privatization and commodification of practically every aspect of human relations, it was in some ways the most profoundly healing aspect of my "restoration."

When I arrived at CIREN, I told my therapist, more in joking bravado than in truth, that I wanted to leave CIREN dancing. On my last day, I waltzed around the entire gym. Nowadays I can go on two-mile hikes with friends, walk fifteen blocks to downtown Berkeley, go to the farmers' market and have a social life. My life is incomparably richer, not only because I'm both more able-bodied and healthier than I've been in years, but because I know in my own flesh that there's another, far more humane way to do medicine.

Will the Real Socialist Medicine Please Stand Up?

Following the health care "debates" from Cuba was surreal. Here the word "socialist" is used to scare people. In Cuba it heals. I spent two months at CIREN, the International Center for Neurological Restoration in Havana, Cuba for treatment of post-stroke weakness, spasticity and pain, a guest of the Cuban people's incredible generosity. I got a variety of therapies for a total of 39 hours a week along with patients from Venezuela, Mexico, Colombia, Portugal, Spain, Italy, Angola and Ukraine. (Cubans are primarily treated at other centers, though I did meet a few at CIREN.) Every day I got four to five hours of physical therapy for my legs and back, two hours of fine motor and upper body work, an hour a day of either holistic medicine (acupuncture mostly) or electric/magnetic field treatments for pain. I also saw a psychologist and a psychiatrist. The only "psychiatric" prescription I was given was for Bach Flower Essences, which are widely used in Cuba. I was also given dental care and saw an allergy specialist.

In Cuba, health care is a human right guaranteed to all Cubans by the constitution, and offered to people in many other countries as an act of humanism and solidarity. In spite of the horrific day-to-day costs of the cruel economic blockade that the US has imposed for fifty years, in spite of dreadful shortages of the most basic supplies (toilet paper, writing paper, soap, pens,) Cubans have continued to prioritize health care and spend a large part of the national budget providing it. And not just any health care.

People come from all over the world for Cuban medicine, not just because it's cheap, but because it's excellent.

Cuban science is not held hostage by corporate sponsorship or the need to create patentable, profitable products. Cuban doctors get their salary from the state, not from a portion of patient costs. There are no insurance companies, and researchers at the Finlay Institute, which developed the vaccine for meningitis B, have also developed effective homeopathic immunizations. Last year one of them prevented an annual epidemic that typically follows hurricane season. It will never make anyone rich. It cost almost nothing to produce. Five million people got the protective dose for free. The Finlay Institute also promotes macrobiotic food, offering classes and a cafeteria where I got all my meals. Cuban doctors are free from the constant threat of lawsuits, which makes them creative, not reckless, and fosters a wonderful climate of open affection, easily expressed in ways that would be considered inappropriate and even grounds for harassment suits in the U.S.

As for me, I went to Cuba in a power wheelchair because I couldn't walk more than 30 to 40 feet, and my arms were too weak for a manual chair. My right hand and foot and my left shoulder gave me nearly constant pain, I got no exercise, had perpetual dark circles under my eyes and was extremely allergic, with two ER crises in the week before my departure.

Now I walk a minimum of ten blocks a day, have full use of my hands and arms, and have only minimal, occasional pain in my right foot. I eat a healthy diet that has cleared my skin and reduced my allergies and I've also lost 20 lbs. which has stabilized my blood sugar, while becoming two centimeters taller. I threw away my sleeping pills and stopped taking a lot of the supplements that were keeping me barely afloat. Every day I take homeopathic formulas for head trauma, hormone balance and detoxification, as well as my flower remedy blend and three cups of turmeric tea, which according to Cuban experts, helps to keep small blood vessels clear of plaque.

When I hear the watered down, pathetic proposals for health care reform being tossed around by our politicians referred to in horrified tones as socialism, as if that's the terrible abyss we must avoid at all cost, I'm clear about whose abyss it is and whose cost.

When right wing fear mongers conjure up pictures of grey faced bureaucrats killing off helpless patients, in an evil empire assembly line of soulless cogs in a cold-hearted machine, I don't think of Hollywood communists, I think of HMO CEOs.

Socialist medicine is about putting human need ahead of greed. Unfortunately, that's not on the table. At least, it's not on the U.S. government's table. When I get furious about the avarice and the lies, when I come home to fourteen insulting pieces of mail from Social Security, placing as many obstacles as possible in the way of my access to Medicare, then I remember the advice of my Cuban psychiatrist about reducing stress and preventing another stroke. Over my cup of turmeric tea I recite her words to myself once more: Increase the level of solidarity in your life. Surround yourself with people who share your values, do important work together, and have fun. And take your flower remedies.

Revolution isn't about radical rhetoric. It's about making societies built on taking care of each other instead of taking advantage of each other. It's about putting human dignity and love above profit, the right to good lives ahead of the right to wealth. This summer I got to live in a revolutionary society —embattled, poor in material resources, bogged down by difficulties, but nevertheless, the most human place I've ever been. So, no, the Obama administration is not proposing socialist medicine, but I am.

Anyone want to share my values, do
important work, and have some fun?

SINS INVALID

The following pieces were written for
Sins Invalid, A performance project of disabled artists,
centering queer artists and artists of color, and exploring
issues of embodiment, sexuality and beauty.

Exoskeleton

My wheelchair is an exoskeleton protecting

the soft body of fatigue.

I get out of bed, walking slowly

on my curved foot and my overworked one;

the foot that cramps and aches and curls inward

onto its edge

trying to figure out where it is, to reconnect,

and the foot that does more than its share and gets tired,

the heroic and sullen foot that steps in to carry the limp.

My whole body aches and trembles with what people call fatigue

as if it had anything to do with a long work week,

a tiresome commute, the ordinary, "boy, I'm bushed!"

of ordinarily tired people.

I carry the fatigue down the stairs to the shed,

unlock the shed, unlock the padlocks,

unplug the recharger cable, slide into the seat,

and suddenly I am uplifted and embraced.

Deep foam cushions me from below and behind.

I am surrounded by the yellow ribs of this new body,

rest my legs on new and stronger bones.

I relax into this enameled-steel-mid-wheeled

statement to the world

that I can't walk another step.

I no longer have to *tell* the people on the buses and trains

to get up out of the specially marked blue symbol seats

because I belong there.

My new outer shell says it for me.

People step aside, apologize for being in my path,

stand without being asked

so I can be strapped into place for my bus ride.

The chair speaks for me,

a new and less exhausting form of speech.

It's the shiny carapace

that lets the world know my species.

I hear they call it being *confined* to a wheelchair.

Before it came, fatigue had me bound tightly to my bed.

When I say fatigue I mean a powdery white sensation,

like silently falling ashes.

I mean an odd, painful tightness all over

as if my skin were shrinking around me.

I mean when the plugs in the arches of my feet

are pulled out

and every ounce of fuel drains away.

I imagine it's my blood

that you can see me turning white as the level drops,

a sinking line of ordinary color like a receding tide.

I mean the fine almost imperceptible tremor of muscles that just can't.

Can't hold a book, lift a glass of water, pick myself up

I mean the trip to the bathroom is a marathon,

something to summon up courage and strength for

and then crawl back onto the bed,

muscles cramping and shaking.

Long before the clenching of a blood vessel in my brain

left the right side of my body confused, noisy, silent, unattached,

wracked with spasms and the searing touch

of nonexistent flame,

I *was* confined.

In the strange world of authorized and unauthorized illness,

it was the stroke

that earned me the right to be believed,

the stroke that lifted me from the bed of exhaustion

into these metal arms, the stroke

that finally brought me the help I needed,

to be carried through the world,

to move without moving,

to fly down the sidewalk the way I fly in dreams,

weaving between people and trees.

I was a housebound invertebrate.

The stroke gave me the right

to purchase these bones.

The stroke set me free.

Drifting to Bottom

I settle into the bed of passive sex like a leaf descending to the bottom of a pond, all of me liquid, languid, slow, luminous, still. Once I was tigerish, licking, biting, pouncing, growling, tumbling, arched, riding the springy rib cages and hips of lovers I could climb on. Now I have sex as plants do, petals agape for pollen; as snails do, one sticky wet part sliding softly, infinitesimally across another. I have sex like a body of water, breath making nipples rise like the crests of waves, creeks emptying into my shimmering state of awareness through crevices, gullies, hillside torrents. Rocking against the coast, tide by tide.

Now I am infinite earth, potent beyond all things, and nearly motionless. Sex is a bead of sweat, dew forming on the curve of a leaf, a thigh. Sex is the quiver of grass on an almost windless day. I am a bed of clay on which your fingers drum like rain, furrowed by your tongue, penetrated by roots that grow strong because of me.

I am the sea anemone, exquisitely sensitive and anchored to rock. My most delicate pink-tipped tentacles suck, clutch, cling to what touches them. I change color, rose to maroon to violet, blush, glow, burn, circle and dance in the water, wrap myself all around what comes within my one inch reach, and never lift myself up from my stony bed. I am held down by tired muscles, topped by my own fatigue, nerve endings tingling with sensations, too exhausted to move, lickable, liquid, languid, sinking into the slick, soft mud, coming down from above, drifting to bottom.

Listen, Speak

1

Come. You. Yes, you. Tonight we are gathering stories, ours, yours. Each of us with our bundles of sticks, each of us with our strands of cord. The word in your pocket is what we need. The song in your heart, the callous on your heel.

Come into the clearing. Bring your tinder. Together, we will strike sparks and set the night ablaze. Come out of the forest, the woodwork, the shadows to this place of freedom, quilombo, swamp town, winter camp, yucayeque, where those not meant to survive laugh and weep together, share breath from mouth to mouth, pass cups of water, break bread—and let our living bodies speak.

Come with your triggers, your losses, your scars. When something you hear, something you see, makes your wounds ache and throb, it's only memory rising, a piece of our history. Bring it into the circle. We will hold it together.

Our history is in our bodies—what we do to breathe, how we move, the sounds we make, our myriad shapes, our wild gestures, far outside the boundaries of what's expected, the knowledge bound into our bones, our trembling muscles, our laboring lungs—like secret seeds tied into the hair of our stolen ancestors, we carry it everywhere. Our stories erupt in the dances we invent, in the pleasure rubbed from our bodies like medicine from crushed leaves, spicy, astringent, sweet.

We are the children of Anacaona, Golden Flower of the Taino, from the lands we called Hayti, Jamayca, Cuba, Boriken, who witnessed the shattering of the Caribbean world, the house of feasting set on fire. A poet warrior speaking truth in a landscape of ashes, speaking beauty into the dark. Though she died at the hands of invaders, we, her descendants, guakía guali, are still here, still speaking unspeakable truths, still making beauty in the marketplace of those who want us dead.

Here come Peg Leg Joe and Moses, the cripple and the epileptic, following their stars across swamps and mountains and cold clear water, saying with their feet, with their backs and hands, no life belongs to another, our bodies are not acreage, livestock, overhead, disposable tools. They hum as they travel, songs heavy with maps that lead us back to ourselves, singing you, yes you, are irreplaceable.

And these are the sterilized multitudes, women of Puerto Rico, one out of three, migrant worker mothers in labor told to sign what they can't read, the poverty-stricken, the weak limbed, the feebleminded, the queer, a poor white girl from Virginia, deemed too stupid to breed, the ones who get migraines, or drink, or like sex, dark skinned, immigrant, colonized, Jew, people like me, people like you...strapped down under surgeons' knives, their bloodlines severed, their children disappeared by stone faced people desperately building a master race to rule the world. Yet here we are, and here we are fruitful, our stories flower, take wing, reproduce like windblown seeds. No surgeon's knife can cut the lines of spirit. Our family tree remains.

2

Open up. Make room. Let the circle grow.

From the shadows steps a man of Tuskeegee, syphilis raging untreated through his veins, gone blind, lame and speechless while white doctors took notes, but here he speaks with a voice like a drum. At the light's edge a girl with no face, who lived ten years locked in a room, holds the hand of an old man with no relatives, and blue numbers tattooed on his arm. Trace the lines in the maps of our bodies. They run like furrows, side by side. They move like rivers, enter each other, make tributaries and forks.

Make room for the children raised on locked wards under a flickering fluorescent light, the shocked and injected, the measured and displayed, tormented, fondled, drugged, called defective. Their small blunt faces look out from sterile hallways, grey buildings, medical case files, toward this fire that we become. They come wheeling and hobbling over thick tree roots, to sit by the flames, cry out in childish voices, for water, for hands to hold, for us to listen as they give themselves new names.

We unwrap our tongues, we bind our stories, we choose to be naked, we show our markings, we lick our fingers, we stroke our bellies, we laugh at midnight, we change the ending, we begin, and begin again.

3

Come beloveds from your narrow places, from your iron beds, from your lonely perches, come warm and sweaty from the arms of lovers, we who invent a world each morning, and speak in fiery tongues.

Come you with voices like seagulls, dissonant and lovely, with hands like roots and twigs. Come limbs that wander and limbs like buds and limbs heavy as stone, come breathless and swollen and weary, fevered and wracked with pain. Come slow and heavy, come wary and scarred, come sweet and harsh and strong. Come arched with pleasure, come slick with honey, come breathless with delight.

You. Yes, you. Take the cord of memory from my hands, and tie a knot to mark your place. Each body knows its own exhausting journey, its own oases of joy, its belly-full of shouting, resilience and shame and jubilation. We mark the trail for each other, put lanterns by the door, scratch our signs in the dirt, make signals with fingers in palms, sing coded freedom songs. Strike the stick of aliveness on whatever will make a sound. Bind your stories together. This is how rope is made. Each strand is essential to the strength of the braid. Bring your body closer. Lean in toward the heat and the light. We are striking sparks of spirit, we are speaking from our flesh, we are stacking up our stories, we are kindling our future.

Listen with your body. Let your body speak.

Aurora Levins Morales

is a Puerto Rican Jewish writer, visual artist, historian and activist. Born in Indiera Baja, Puerto Rico in 1954, she has lived most of her life with chronic illness and disability. This collection of writings on the body, and the experience and politics of illness and medicine, was assembled in January, 2013 to raise funds for her ongoing health care needs, following a medical crisis involving bulging discs, pinched nerves, and dependency on narcotic pain medications.

**Proceeds from the sale of this book
will pay for medical and attendant care.**

For updates on Aurora's condition,
or to donate to her health
care fund, see:

www.auroralevinsmorales.com

Also by Aurora Levins Morales:

Getting Home Alive
(with Rosario Morales), Firebrand Books, 1986

Revised & Expanded Edition coming in 2014 from Palabrera Press

This mother–daughter, mixed genre collaboration was hailed as "a landmark in US Puerto Rican literature" and "the most important book to come out of the diaspora in a generation," a call and response across generations, migration and languages.

"Serious, literary and passionate." — Publisher's Weekly

Medicine Stories
South End Press, 1998

In Medicine Stories, Levins Morales writes lucidly about the complexities of social identity. Her lyrical meditations on ecology, children's liberation, sexuality, and history show how political transformation and personal healing are inextricably bound. Levins Morales is a survivor of childhood sexual abuse and was raised as a Jewish "red diaper baby" in the mountains of Puerto Rico.

At the heart of this book is the conviction that our survival depends on crafting a political practice capable of healing all our wounds, from global, macro-economic injustices to the intimate scars of cruelty in our own lives.

Remedios: Stories Of Earth And Iron From The History Of Puertorriqueñas

Beacon Press 1998 / South End Press 2001

"Captivating language and enticing cadence are characteristics of the enchanting prose Levins Morales employs in this gathering of uniquely realized vignettes...Exciting melange of stories ultimately affirming the empowerment of women."

— Booklist

"There is no other book like Remedios. It is history, anthropology, poetry, and myth; it is a song and a prayer. Aurora Levins Morales is a Jewish Latina curandera who embraces diverse legacies with passion and eloquence. In stories so beautifully told they soar off the page...she offers us remedies that heal our bodies and souls and feed our spirits of our many forgotten ancestors."

—Ruth Behar, author of The Vulnerable Observer

Telling To Live: Latina Feminist Testimonios

By The Latina Feminist Group, Duke University Press, 2001

"Telling to Live may be one of the most important books published in the last few decades. Latinas collectively have not had a book like this before that features so many different backgrounds and cultures...The inclusion of all these mix-and-match identifications is what makes this book required reading in women's studies classes all across the globe."

—Jocelyn Climent, in Bust

Coming soon from Palabrera Press:

Coming in Fall 2013

Poet On Assignment

Following 9/11 Aurora Levins Morales' poem "Shema" went viral. It was repeatedly broadcast on Pacifica radio, and read at dozens of anti-war demonstrations nationwide. During the following months, Aurora was hired by Pacifica's Flashpoints news magazine to write poetry commentaries on the news. Poet On Assignment collects these "rapid response poems" for the first time. With an introduction by Flashpoints producer Dennis Bernstein.

Coming in 2014

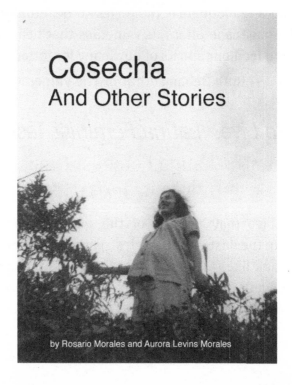

Cosecha
And Other Stories

by Rosario Morales and Aurora Levins Morales

Cosecha and Other Stories

25 years after the publication of their ground breaking mixed-genre book Getting Home Alive, Palabrera Press presents another mother-daughter collaboration by Rosario Morales and Aurora Levins Morales.

"She was an excellent hostess, thoughtful, self-effacing and nurturing. Pale young lawyers, mustachioed cultural gurus, callow revolutionaries, mathematical near geniuses, and multicolored social butterflies of all sexes lunged against her upholstered furniture and hand woven pillows, amongst her statuettes and doilies, drinking, sneering, laughing, shouting, eating, necking, destroying reputations, puncturing egos and generally enjoying themselves. She moved softly among them, extinguishing cigarettes, replenishing drinks, re-refilling plates, extracting stilettos, applying band-aids, and restoring shoes, unseen and unheard."
— from "Unseen" by Rosario

"Nights while the stars swung overhead we leaned in slow, delicious free fall toward each other's arms, knowing we would arrive in our own good time. Apples, berries, nuts, pumpkins, late corn all spilled their abundance from the roadside stands. Around us the trees glowed in the colors of sun-ripe fruit, flickering and bright as faces turned to a hidden fire. But all the time the roots were reaching for a place deeper than the approaching frost, a race against the tilt of the earth's axis."
— from "First Snow" by Aurora

Made in United States
North Haven, CT
26 November 2023

44573313R00114